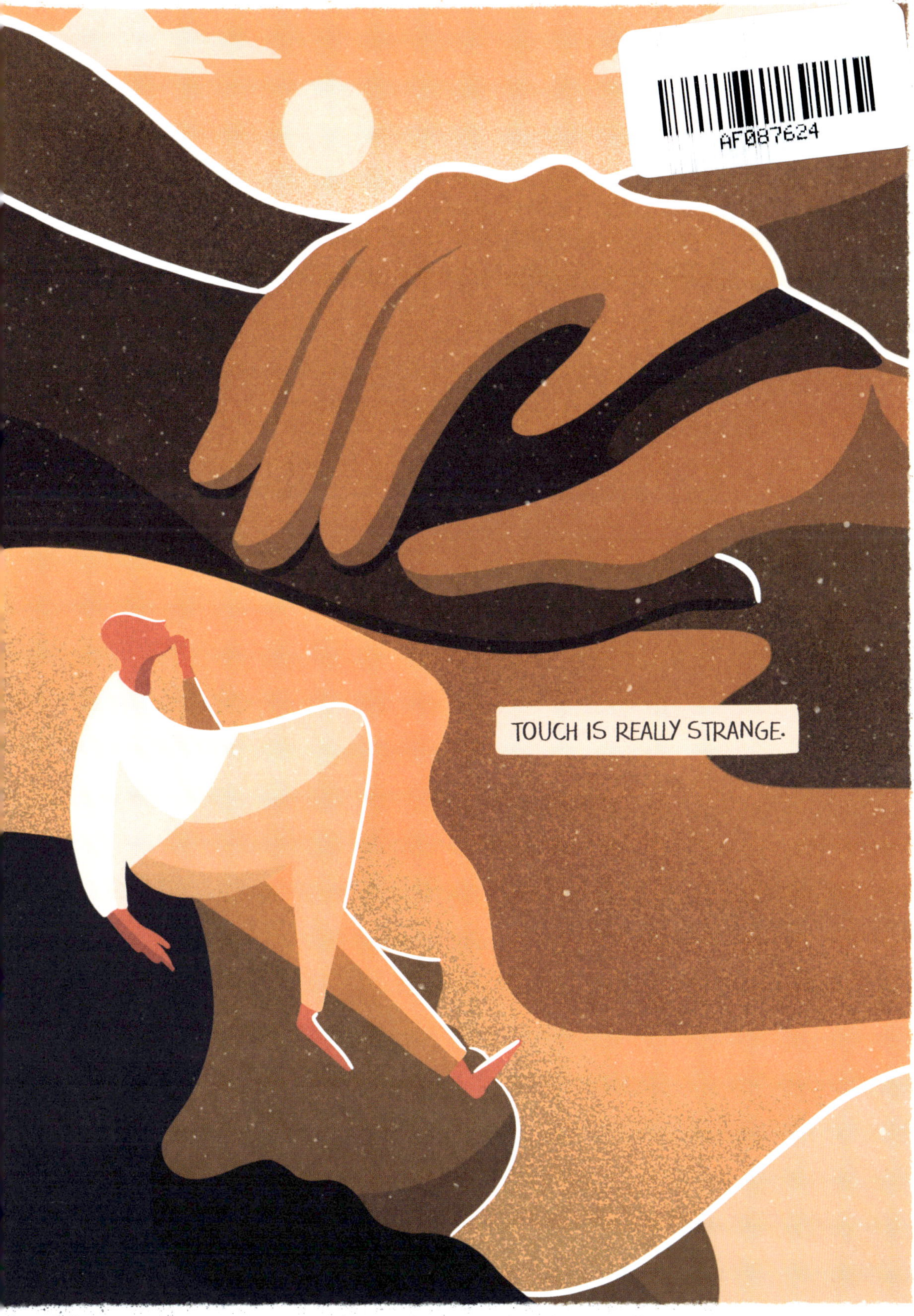
TOUCH IS REALLY STRANGE.

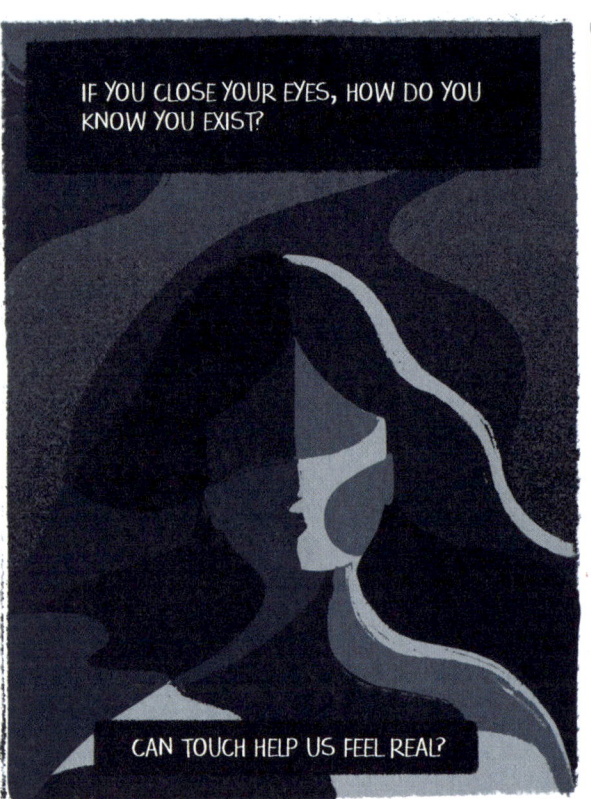
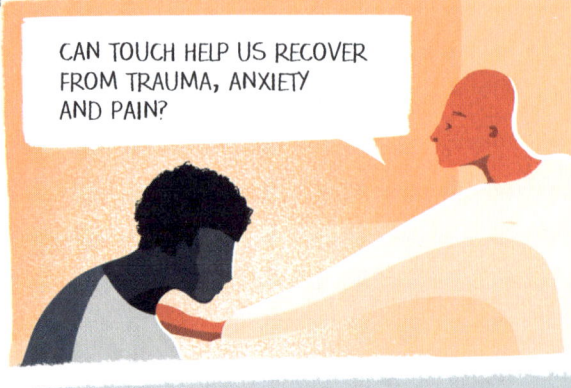
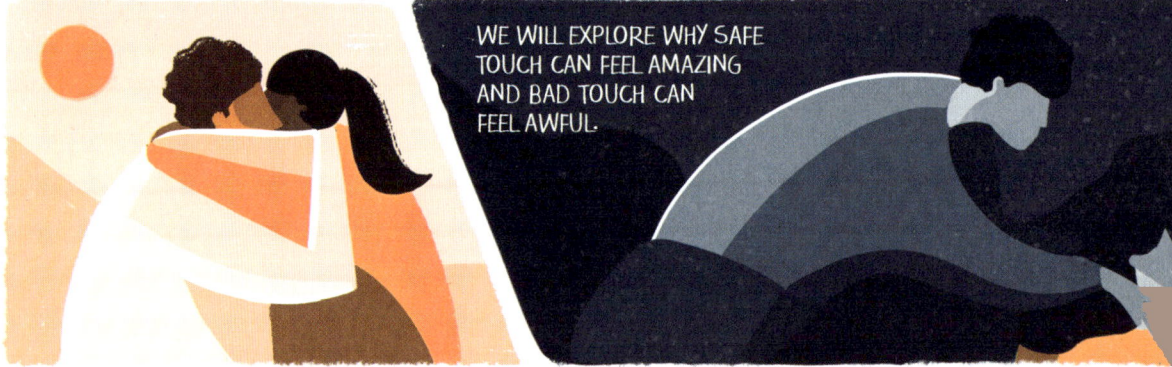
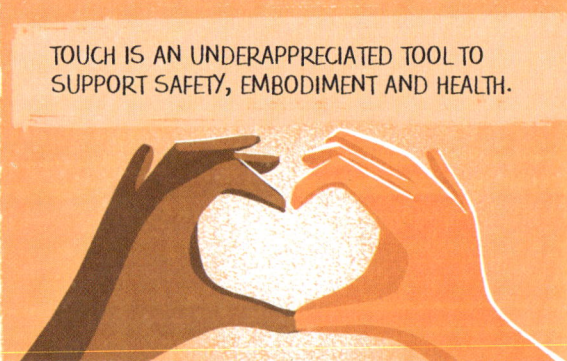

Margaret Atwood (2000) beautifully captures the importance of touch: 'Touch comes before sight, before speech. It is the first language and the last and it always tells the truth.' Touch is our earliest sense to develop: 'Touch is thought to become functional in utero, at about 8 weeks' (Linden 2015).

'It is not enough to read that the sand on the beach is soft, I want my bare feet to feel it. I have no use for any knowledge that is not preceded by a sensation' (Gide 1895). 'Touch is one of the most essential elements of human development...and a powerful healing force' (Zur and Nordmarken 2020).

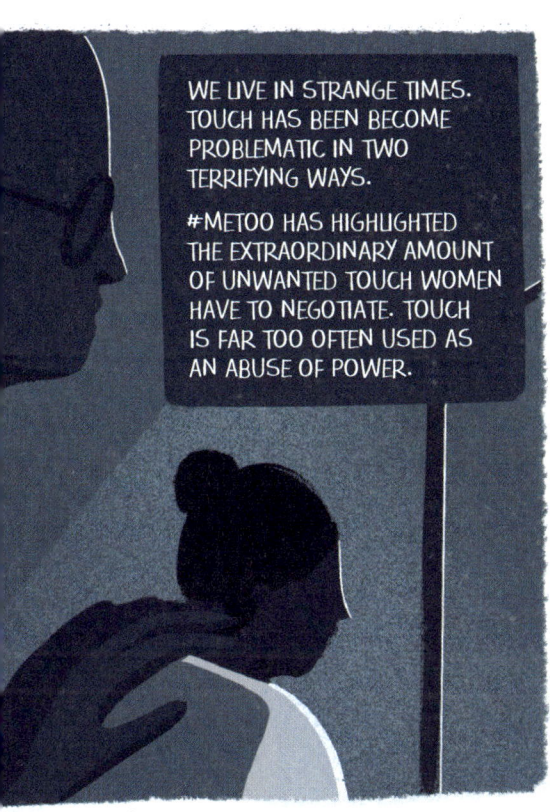

WE LIVE IN STRANGE TIMES. TOUCH HAS BEEN BECOME PROBLEMATIC IN TWO TERRIFYING WAYS.

#METOO HAS HIGHLIGHTED THE EXTRAORDINARY AMOUNT OF UNWANTED TOUCH WOMEN HAVE TO NEGOTIATE. TOUCH IS FAR TOO OFTEN USED AS AN ABUSE OF POWER.

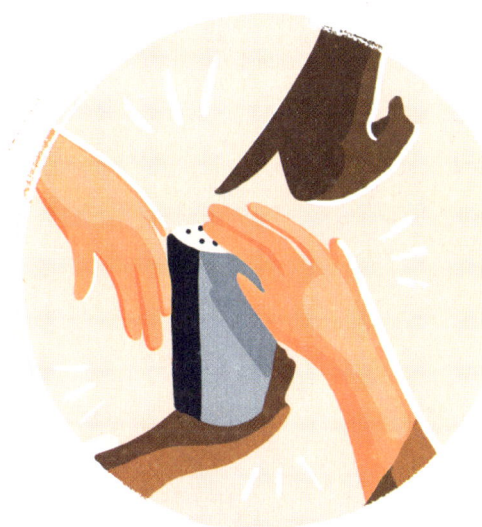

COVID-19 HAS TURNED A GESTURE THAT HAS BEEN COMMON FOR HUNDREDS OF YEARS – SHAKING HANDS – INTO AN ACT OF CONTAGION. TOUCHING PEOPLE, TOUCHING BUTTONS, TOUCHING SALT SHAKERS – BASICALLY TOUCHING ANYTHING SHARED – IS NOW A RISKY ACTIVITY.

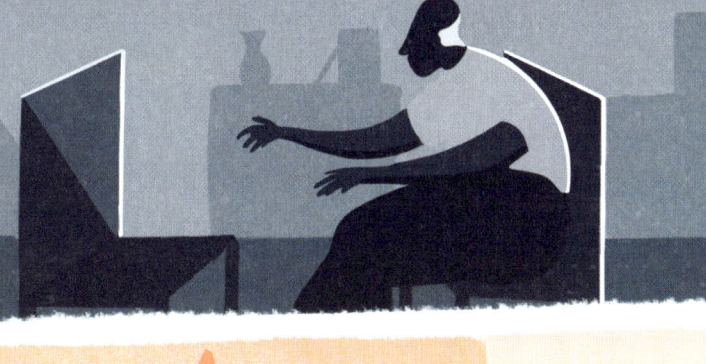

HOWEVER, A CONSISTENT LAMENT DURING LOCKDOWN WAS THAT THE LACK OF HUGS AND HUMAN CONTACT WAS PROFOUNDLY FELT.

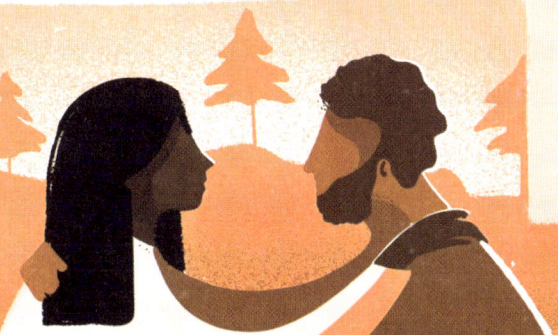

SO, IN SPITE OF THE FEARS AROUND TOUCH, DEEP DOWN WE UNDERSTAND THAT IT IS OF FUNDAMENTAL IMPORTANCE.

READ ON TO CELEBRATE AND LEARN HOW TOUCH WORKS AND HOW 'RELATIONAL TOUCH' CAN BE A FORCE FOR GOOD.

Pre-COVID-19, researchers argued that the skill of touch had faded. Tiffany Field stated in 2001, 'American society is dangerously touch deprived.' 'A worker turned to a colleague and asked to borrow the salt. As well as the saltshaker, in that instant, they shared the new coronavirus' (Reuters 2020).

'How do we live with this unbearable skin hunger?' 'I cannot wait to have my hair washed at my hairdresser. ... Her hands are delicious and confident and kind, equally firm and gentle.' V (formerly Eve Ensler 2020) beautifully explores lack of touch in lockdown.

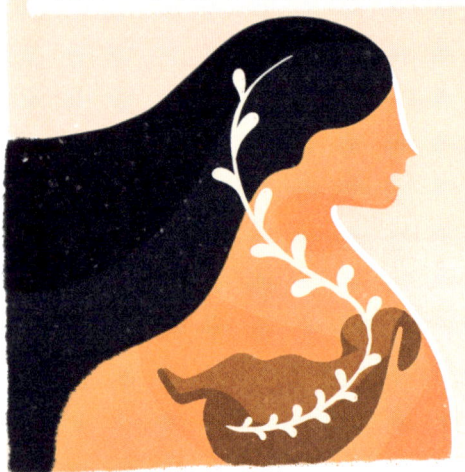

LET'S LOOK AT THE POWER OF TOUCH.

SKIN-TO-SKIN CONTACT IS NOW UNIVERSALLY RECOMMENDED TO HELP BABIES THRIVE.

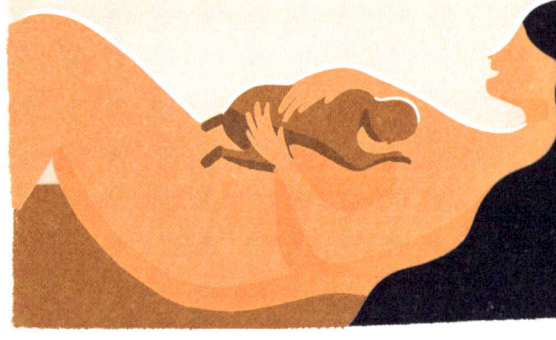

IT CALMS AND RELAXES BOTH MOTHER AND BABY, REGULATES THE BABY'S HEART RATE AND BREATHING, AND REDUCES STRESS.

'KANGAROO CARE', WHERE THE BABY IS HELD AGAINST THE BARE CHEST, SAVES PRE-TERM BABIES' LIVES.

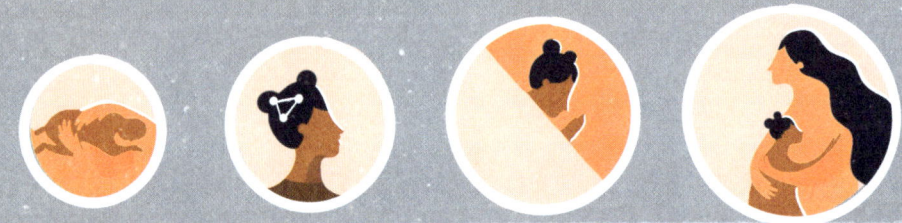

BENEFITS OF SKIN-TO-SKIN CONTACT ARE KNOWN TO EXTEND INTO LATER LIFE: AT 10, CHILDREN ARE LESS STRESSED, SLEEP BETTER AND ARE MORE ATTUNED.

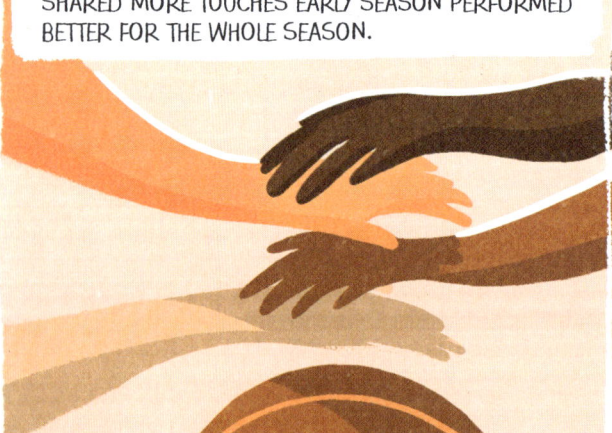

TOUCH IS SOCIAL GLUE. BASKETBALL TEAMS THAT SHARED MORE TOUCHES EARLY SEASON PERFORMED BETTER FOR THE WHOLE SEASON.

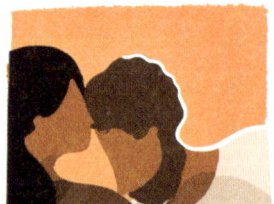 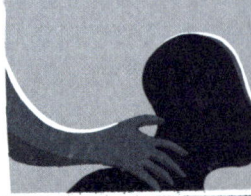

EVERYDAY GESTURES, SUCH AS A PAT ON THE BACK OR A CARESS OF THE ARM, ARE 'FAR MORE PROFOUND THAN WE USUALLY REALIZE'. TOUCH 'IS THE PRIMARY LANGUAGE OF COMPASSION, LOVE, AND GRATITUDE'.

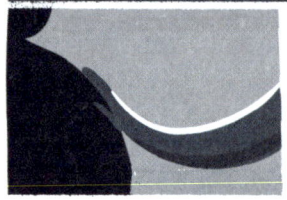 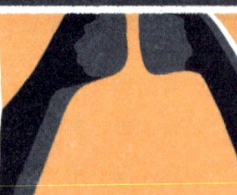

'When a mother holds her baby in skin to skin contact after birth it initiates strong instinctive behaviours in both' (UNICEF 2019). 'Children receiving Kangaroo Care showed attenuated stress response, improved respiratory sinus arrhythmia, organized sleep, and better cognitive control' (Feldman et al. 2014).

'Interpersonal touch is a crucial form of social glue.' For NBA players, 'celebratory touch...was associated with higher performance' (Linden 2015). Dacher Keltner (2009), an influential emotion researcher, is the source for the touch and compassion quotes.

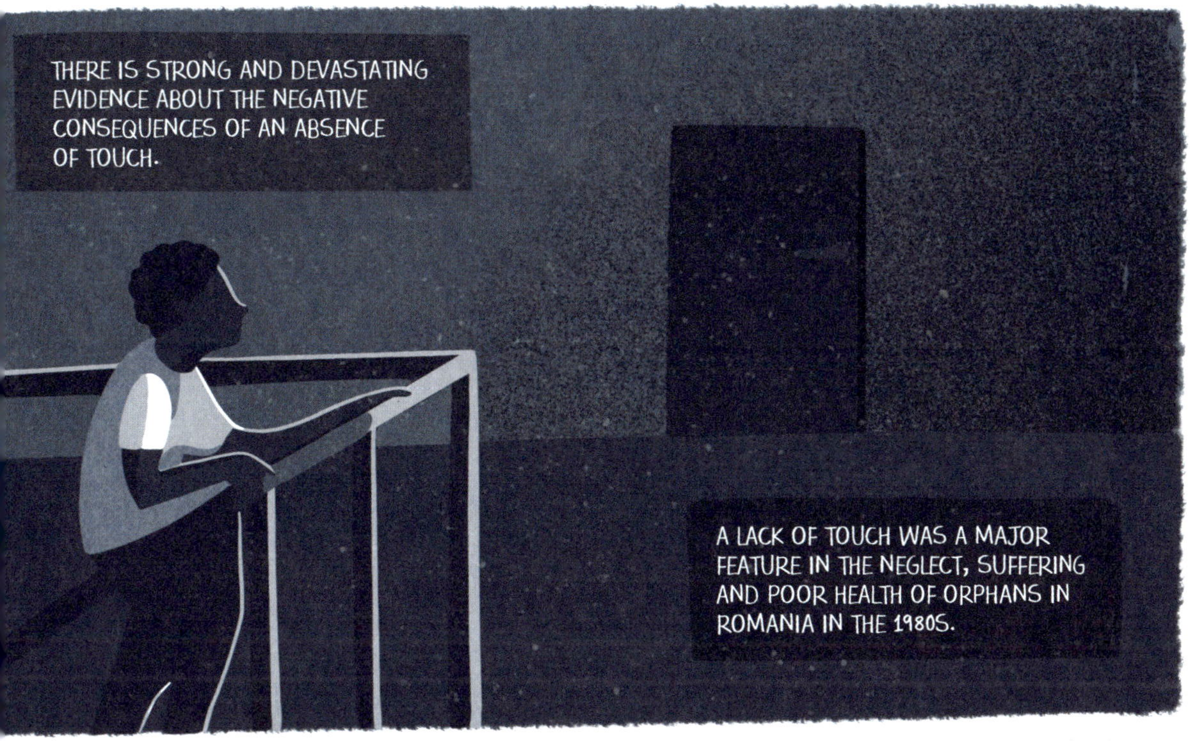

THERE IS STRONG AND DEVASTATING EVIDENCE ABOUT THE NEGATIVE CONSEQUENCES OF AN ABSENCE OF TOUCH.

A LACK OF TOUCH WAS A MAJOR FEATURE IN THE NEGLECT, SUFFERING AND POOR HEALTH OF ORPHANS IN ROMANIA IN THE 1980S.

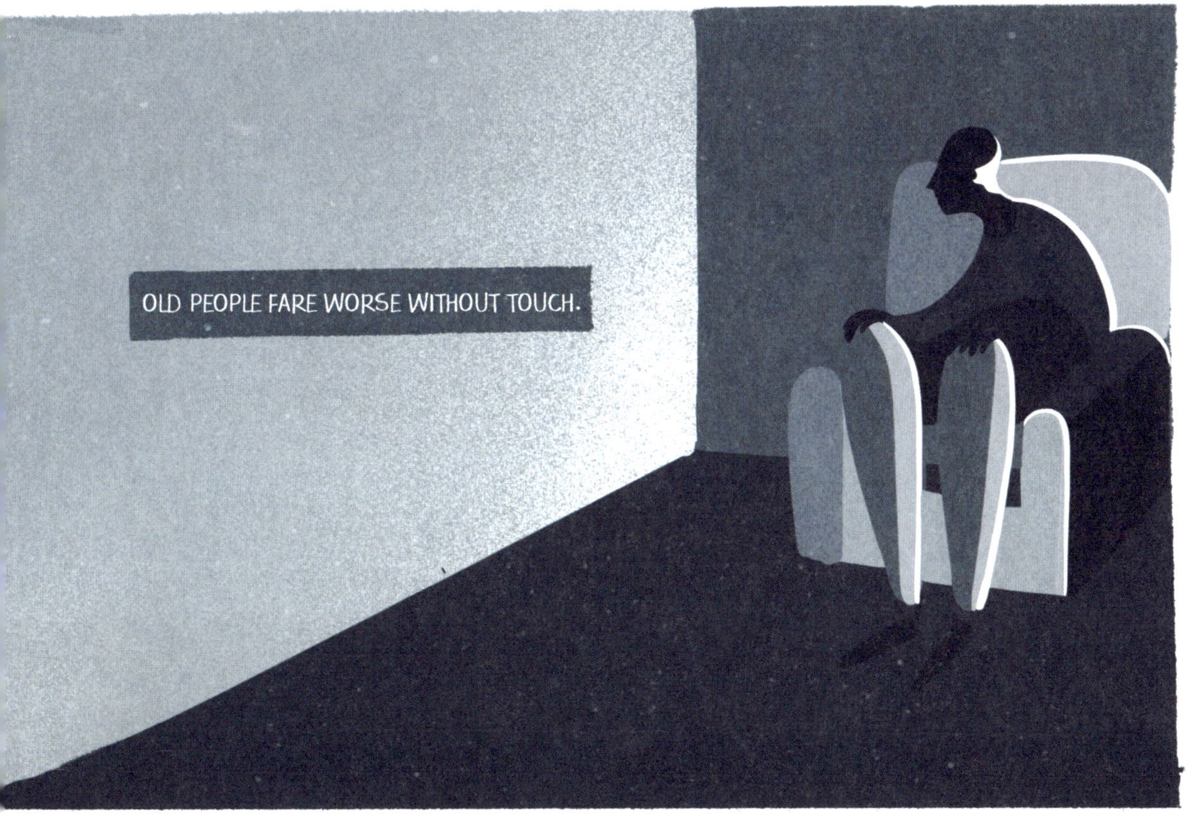

OLD PEOPLE FARE WORSE WITHOUT TOUCH.

'Children without touch, stimulation, and nurturing can literally lose the capacity to form any meaningful relationships for the rest of their lives.' 'The role of touch and sensory input in attachment is paramount and includes holding, rocking, feeding, gazing, and physical proximity' (Courtney and Nolan 2017).

'An absence of human touch can cause negative physical and emotional effects for older adults. Without human touch, elders are at increased risk of anxiety, feeling isolated, lowered trust in care partners and decreased awareness of the senses' (Elder Care Alliance 2017).

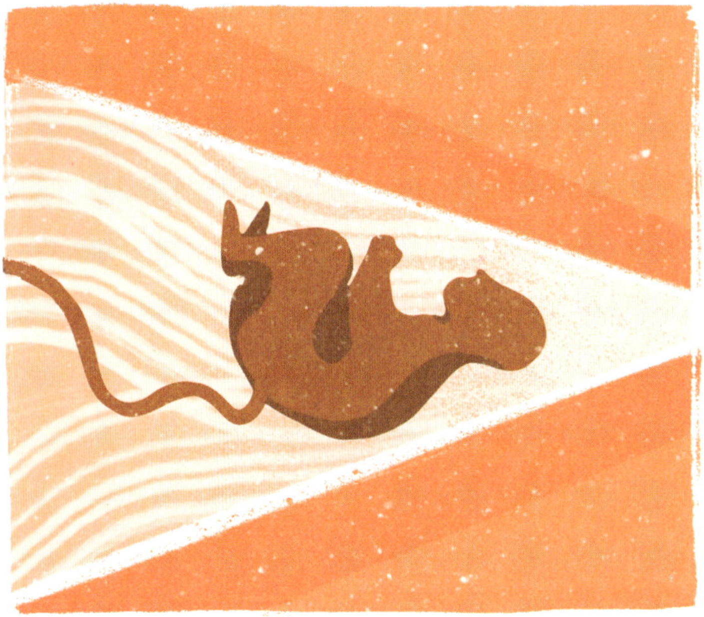

OUR FIRST EXPERIENCES ARE ALL BASED ON TOUCH.

PASSING THROUGH THE BIRTH CANAL IS PROBABLY ONE OF THE HARDEST THINGS WE EVER DID. THERE IS PUSHING, RESISTANCE, THE RIGHT SUPPORT OR THE NEED TO FIND OUR OWN WAY.

THE FORCES WE EXPERIENCED WILL CALIBRATE OUR THREAT DETECTION SYSTEMS AS TO WHAT IS TOO QUICK, TOO SLOW, TOO HARD, TOO MUCH.

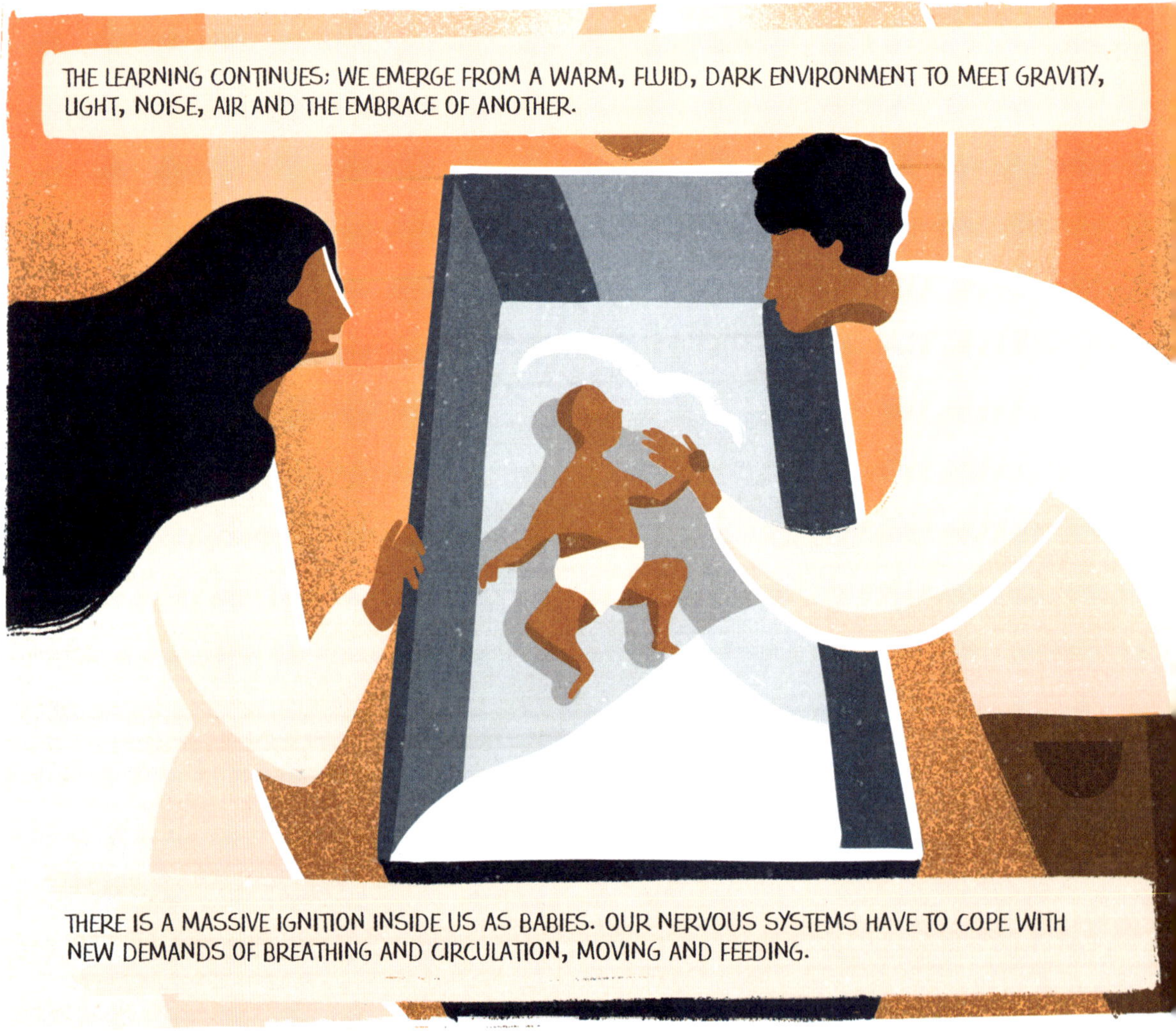
THE LEARNING CONTINUES; WE EMERGE FROM A WARM, FLUID, DARK ENVIRONMENT TO MEET GRAVITY, LIGHT, NOISE, AIR AND THE EMBRACE OF ANOTHER.
THERE IS A MASSIVE IGNITION INSIDE US AS BABIES. OUR NERVOUS SYSTEMS HAVE TO COPE WITH NEW DEMANDS OF BREATHING AND CIRCULATION, MOVING AND FEEDING.

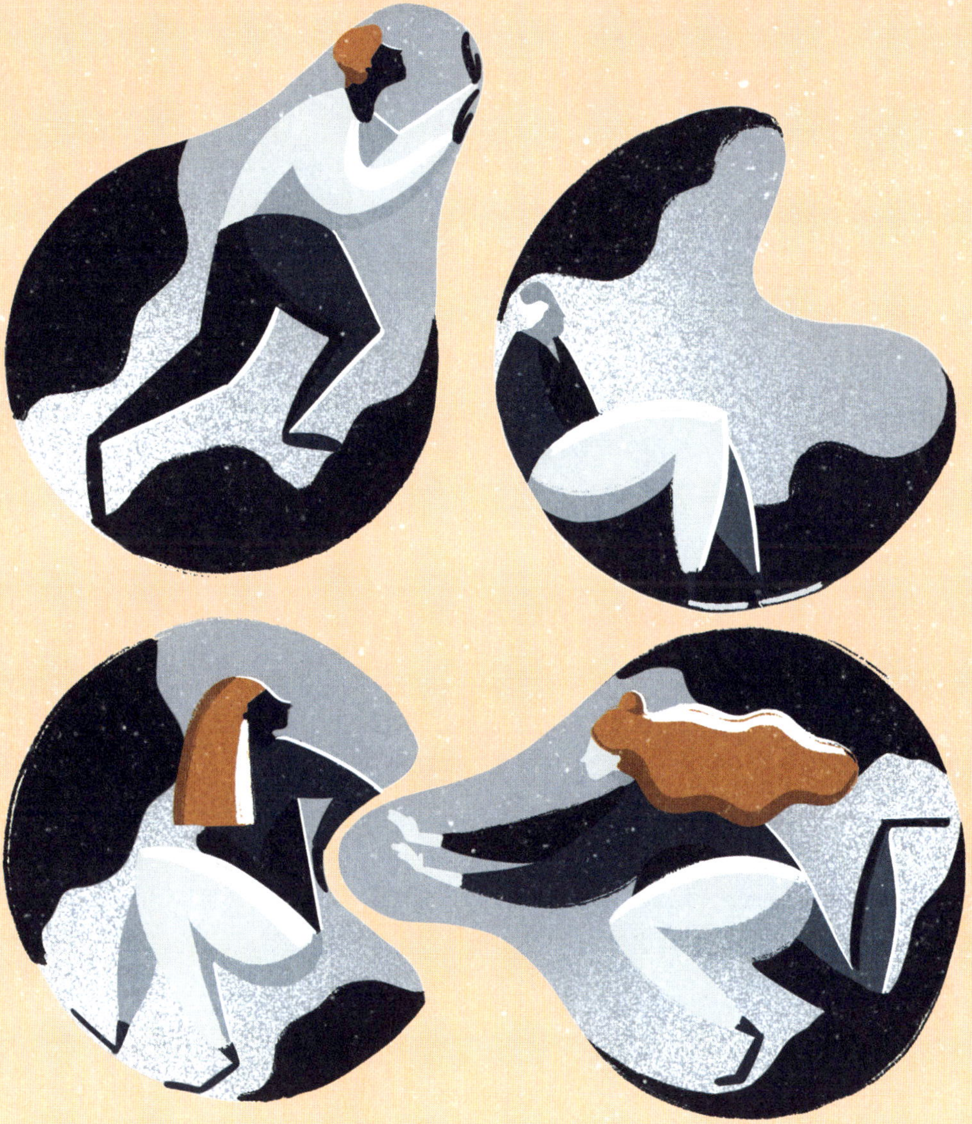

ALL LEARNING IS ROOTED IN OUR INITIAL EXPERIENCES OF PHYSICAL INTERACTION WITH A WORLD THAT IMPRESSES ITSELF UPON US. WE PUSH AGAINST THINGS AND THEY PUSH BACK. WE FIND OUR EDGES AND OUR SENSE OF WHAT WE CAN CONTROL, WHAT HELPS AND WHAT HINDERS.

WHEN THE WORLD PUSHED BACK, IT MAY NOT ALWAYS HAVE BEEN GENTLE. IF WE ARE LUCKY, WE FIND ENOUGH SAFETY, SUCH THAT NOVELTY CONTINUES TO BE EXCITING RATHER THAN SOMETHING TO BE FEARED.

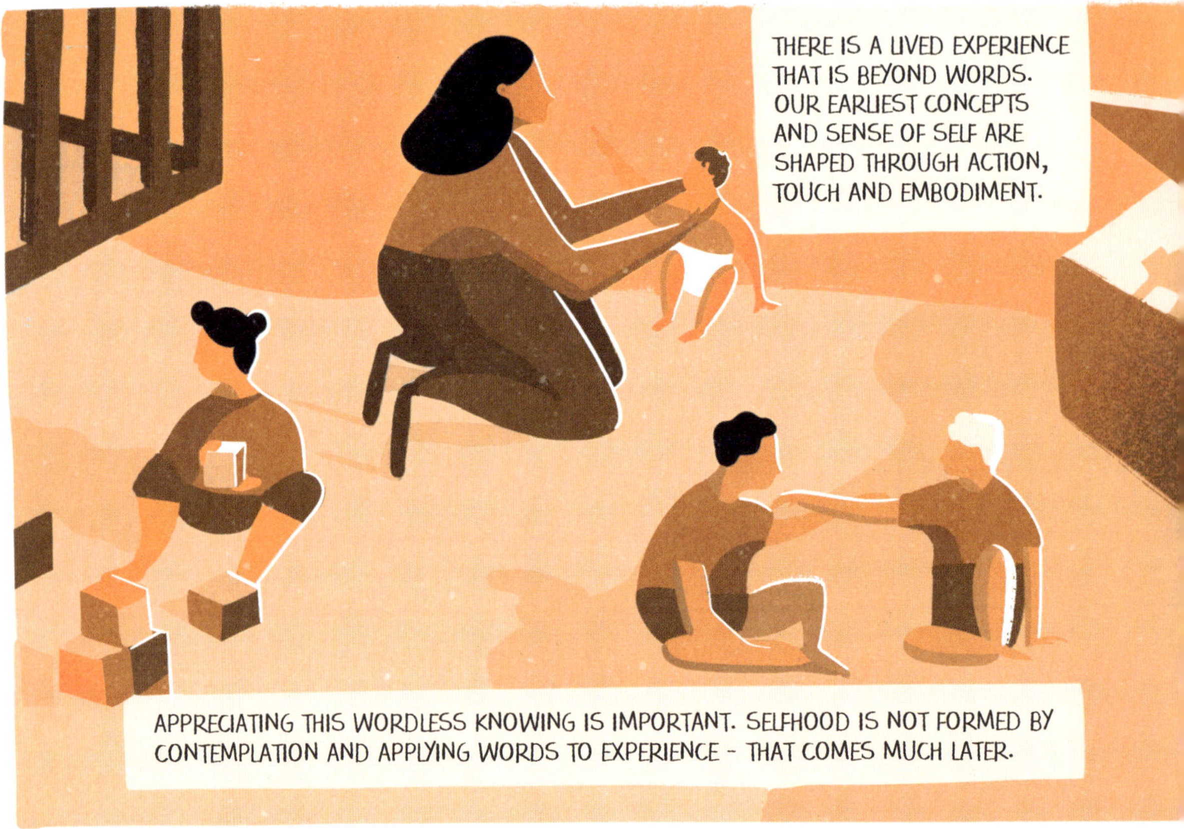

THERE IS A LIVED EXPERIENCE THAT IS BEYOND WORDS. OUR EARLIEST CONCEPTS AND SENSE OF SELF ARE SHAPED THROUGH ACTION, TOUCH AND EMBODIMENT.

APPRECIATING THIS WORDLESS KNOWING IS IMPORTANT. SELFHOOD IS NOT FORMED BY CONTEMPLATION AND APPLYING WORDS TO EXPERIENCE - THAT COMES MUCH LATER.

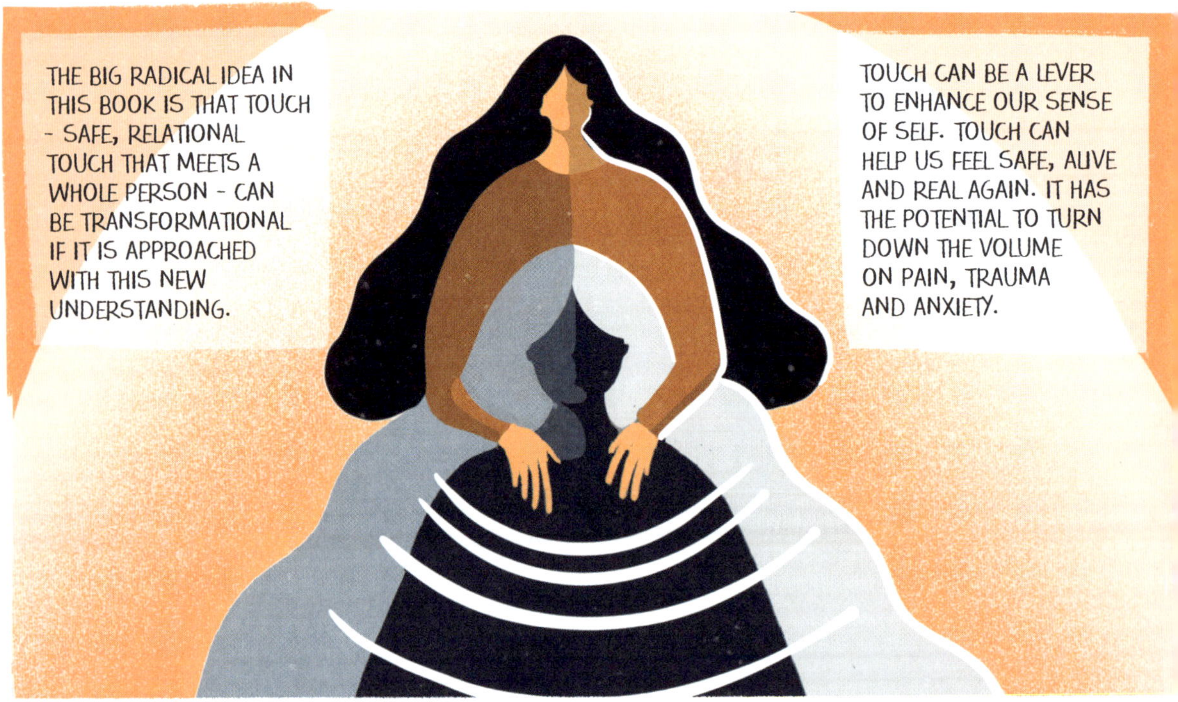

THE BIG RADICAL IDEA IN THIS BOOK IS THAT TOUCH - SAFE, RELATIONAL TOUCH THAT MEETS A WHOLE PERSON - CAN BE TRANSFORMATIONAL IF IT IS APPROACHED WITH THIS NEW UNDERSTANDING.

TOUCH CAN BE A LEVER TO ENHANCE OUR SENSE OF SELF. TOUCH CAN HELP US FEEL SAFE, ALIVE AND REAL AGAIN. IT HAS THE POTENTIAL TO TURN DOWN THE VOLUME ON PAIN, TRAUMA AND ANXIETY.

'All perception is touch-like... Think of a blind person tap-tapping his or her way around a cluttered space, perceiving that space by touch, not all at once, but through time, by skilful probing and movement. The world makes itself available to the perceiver through physical movement and interaction' (Noë 2006).

Use of our body from birth creates patterns that 'are embodied and give coherent, meaningful structure to our physical experience at a preconceptual level' (Johnson 1987). We know our body 'primarily through the various tactile sensations involved in any activity of touching something' (Welton 1999, quoting Husserl).

HUMANS ARE RESTLESS, QUIVERING, PULSING ORGANISMS. WE ARE SELF-ORGANIZING AGENTS THAT EVOLVED TO EXPLORE.

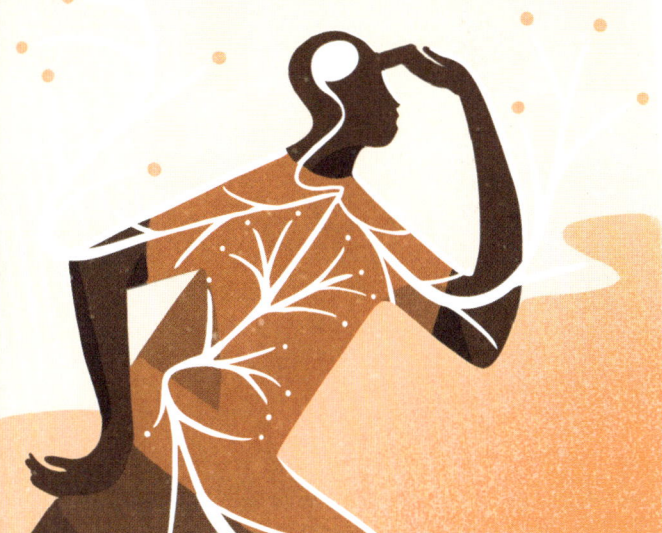

WE INHERENTLY SEEK NOVELTY. TO BE CREATIVE AND PLAYFUL, TO REACH FOR WHAT IS BEYOND THE HORIZON, IS A DEEP DRIVE IN OUR PHYSIOLOGY. VARIETY AND THE RIGHT AMOUNT OF CHALLENGE PROMOTE GROWTH.

THE OPPOSITE IS CONTRACTION, FEAR AND MOVING AWAY. THIS CAN BE FELT IN THE GESTURES, POSTURES AND MOVEMENTS WE MAKE. THERE IS AN ASSOCIATED WITHDRAWAL INTO PRIVATE, UNTOUCHABLE, MENTAL WORLDS.

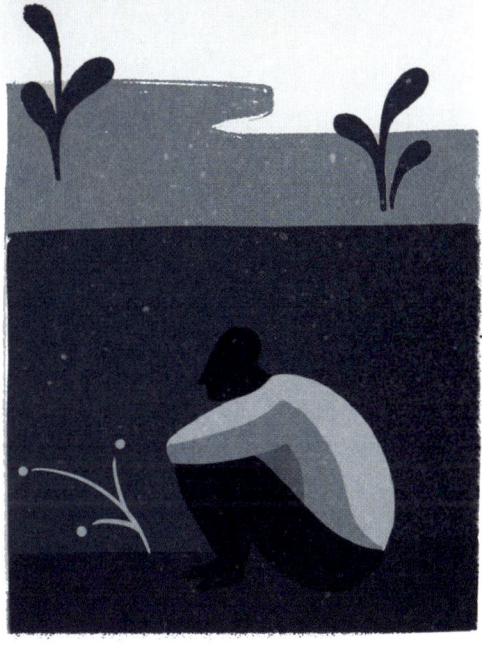

'ACTION MOULDS PERCEPTION.' PROFESSOR BARBARA TVERSKY REINFORCES THE IDEA THAT HOW WE ACT AND INTERACT SHAPES HOW WE FEEL.

'OUR PERCEPTION AND UNDERSTANDING OF THE BODIES OF OTHERS ARE DEEPLY CONNECTED TO THE ACTIONS AND SENSATIONS OF OUR OWN BODIES.'

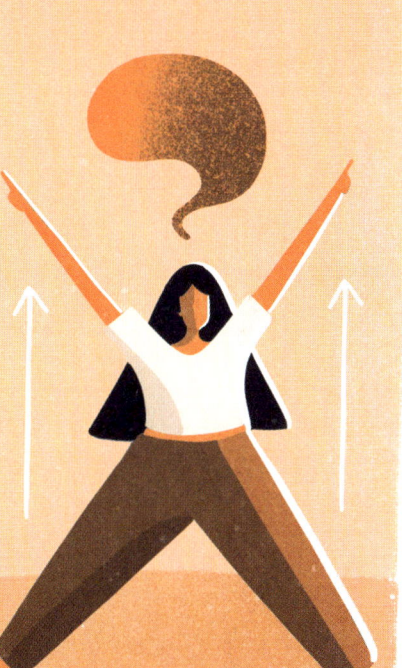

WE MOVE, WE TOUCH, WE EXPLORE SPACE. THESE ARE THE FOUNDATIONS OF THOUGHT.

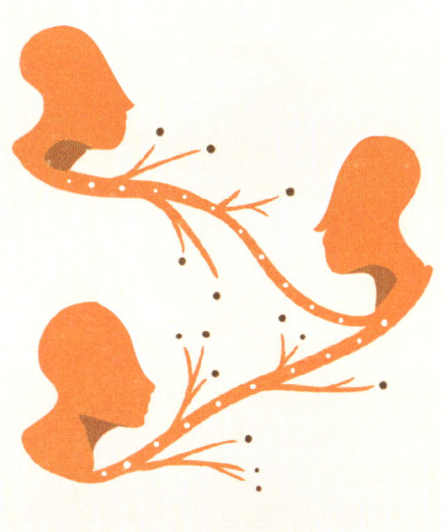

Jessica Riskin (2016) on agency: 'I mean something like consciousness but more basic, more rudimentary, a primitive, prerequisite quality...an intrinsic capacity to act in the world.' Emotion researcher Jaak Panksepp (2010) stated '"Seeking" or "avoidance" are the fundamental goals of brain activity.'

'Rhythm is deeply embedded in our bodies, in our hearts, our breathing, our brains, our actions... Our rhythms organize and synchronize our bodies...and synchronize our bodies with the bodies of others.' 'Movement and our interactions in space, not language, are the true foundation of thought' (Tversky 2019).

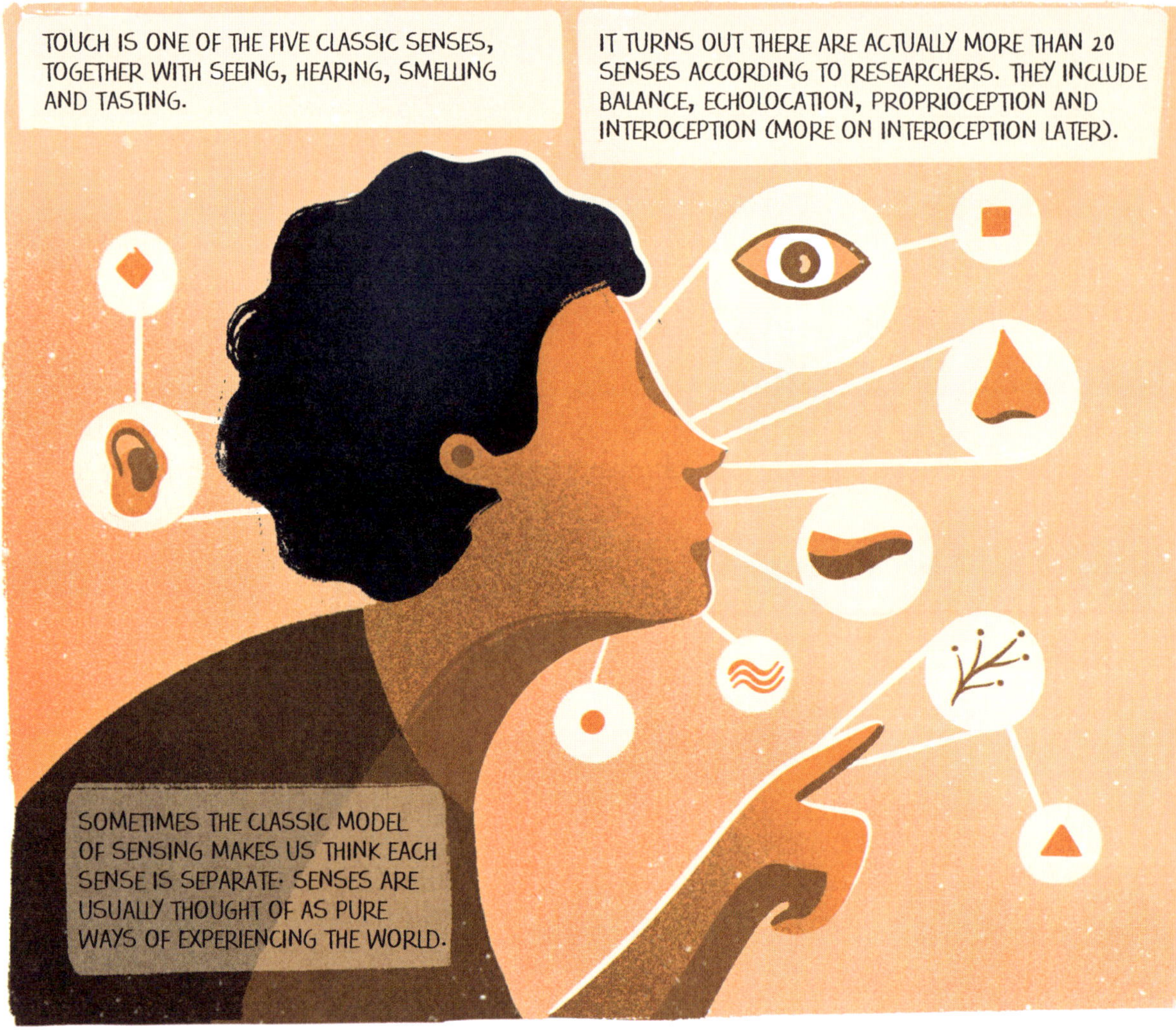
TOUCH IS ONE OF THE FIVE CLASSIC SENSES, TOGETHER WITH SEEING, HEARING, SMELLING AND TASTING.
IT TURNS OUT THERE ARE ACTUALLY MORE THAN 20 SENSES ACCORDING TO RESEARCHERS. THEY INCLUDE BALANCE, ECHOLOCATION, PROPRIOCEPTION AND INTEROCEPTION (MORE ON INTEROCEPTION LATER).
SOMETIMES THE CLASSIC MODEL OF SENSING MAKES US THINK EACH SENSE IS SEPARATE. SENSES ARE USUALLY THOUGHT OF AS PURE WAYS OF EXPERIENCING THE WORLD.

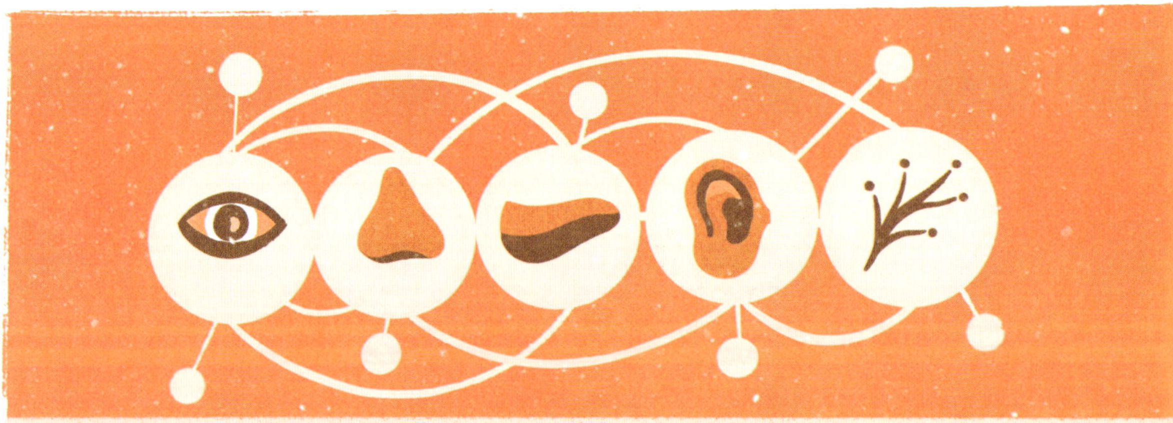

HOWEVER, ALL THESE MODES OF SENSING ARE INTEGRATED TOGETHER TO SERVE THE GOALS OF THE BRAIN. THE CONTEXT AND COMPETING PRIORITIES INSIDE US COLOUR ALL MODES OF PERCEPTION.

'There is, in fact, no pure touch sensation, for by the time we have perceived a touch, it has been blended with other sensory input, plans for action, expectations, and a healthy dose of emotion' (Linden 2015). This is true for all senses. 'The sense we rely on most for reality is touch' (Smith 2018).

Touch is 'inherently multisensory' and 'cannot be associated solely with the skin in any simplistic way'. 'Touch seems to require active exploratory movements' and has a 'close connection to agency'. 'Only in touch do we seem to come into direct contact with reality' (Fulkerson 2020).

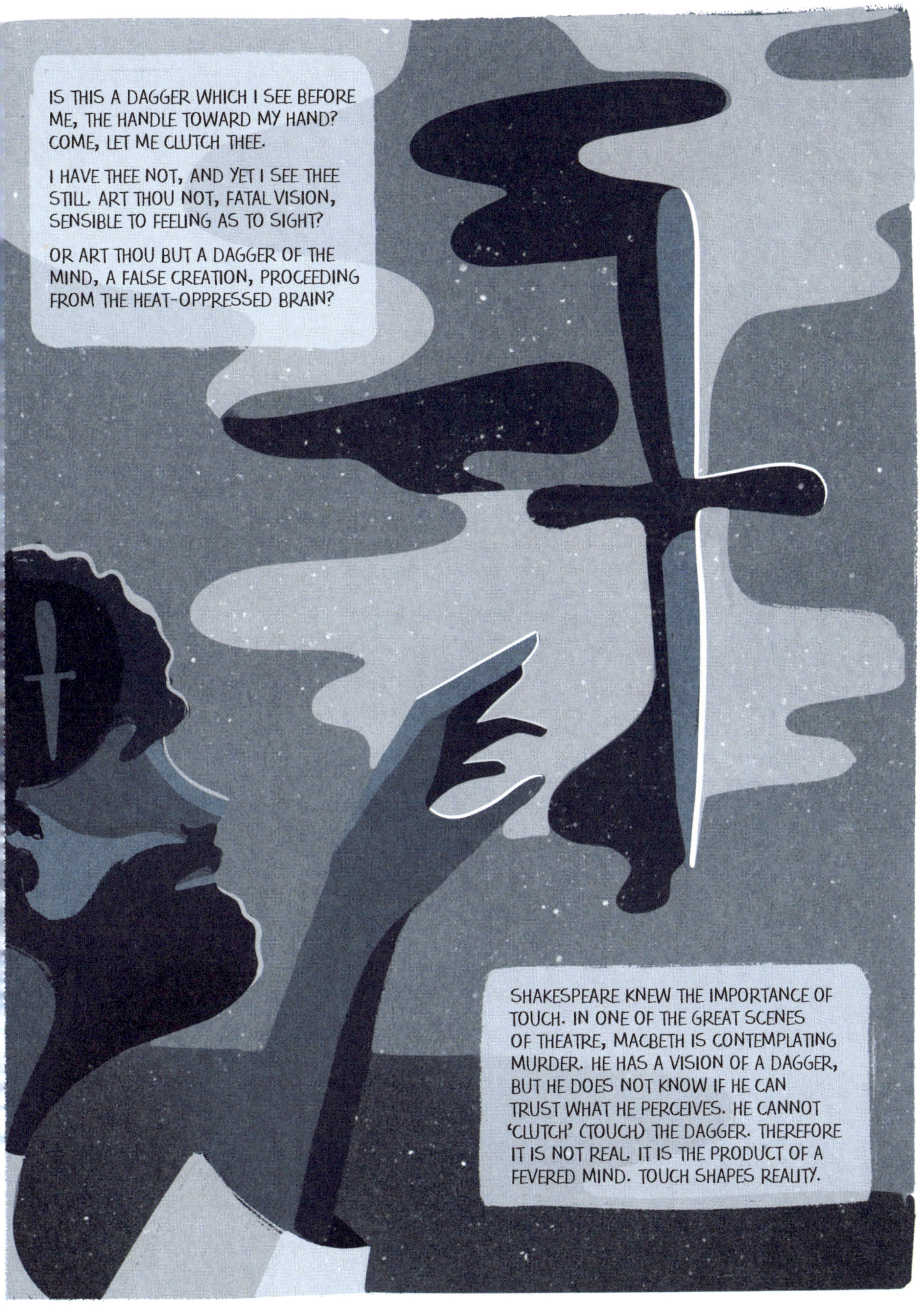
IS THIS A DAGGER WHICH I SEE BEFORE ME, THE HANDLE TOWARD MY HAND? COME, LET ME CLUTCH THEE.
I HAVE THEE NOT, AND YET I SEE THEE STILL. ART THOU NOT, FATAL VISION, SENSIBLE TO FEELING AS TO SIGHT?
OR ART THOU BUT A DAGGER OF THE MIND, A FALSE CREATION, PROCEEDING FROM THE HEAT-OPPRESSED BRAIN?
SHAKESPEARE KNEW THE IMPORTANCE OF TOUCH. IN ONE OF THE GREAT SCENES OF THEATRE, MACBETH IS CONTEMPLATING MURDER. HE HAS A VISION OF A DAGGER, BUT HE DOES NOT KNOW IF HE CAN TRUST WHAT HE PERCEIVES. HE CANNOT 'CLUTCH' (TOUCH) THE DAGGER. THEREFORE IT IS NOT REAL. IT IS THE PRODUCT OF A FEVERED MIND. TOUCH SHAPES REALITY.

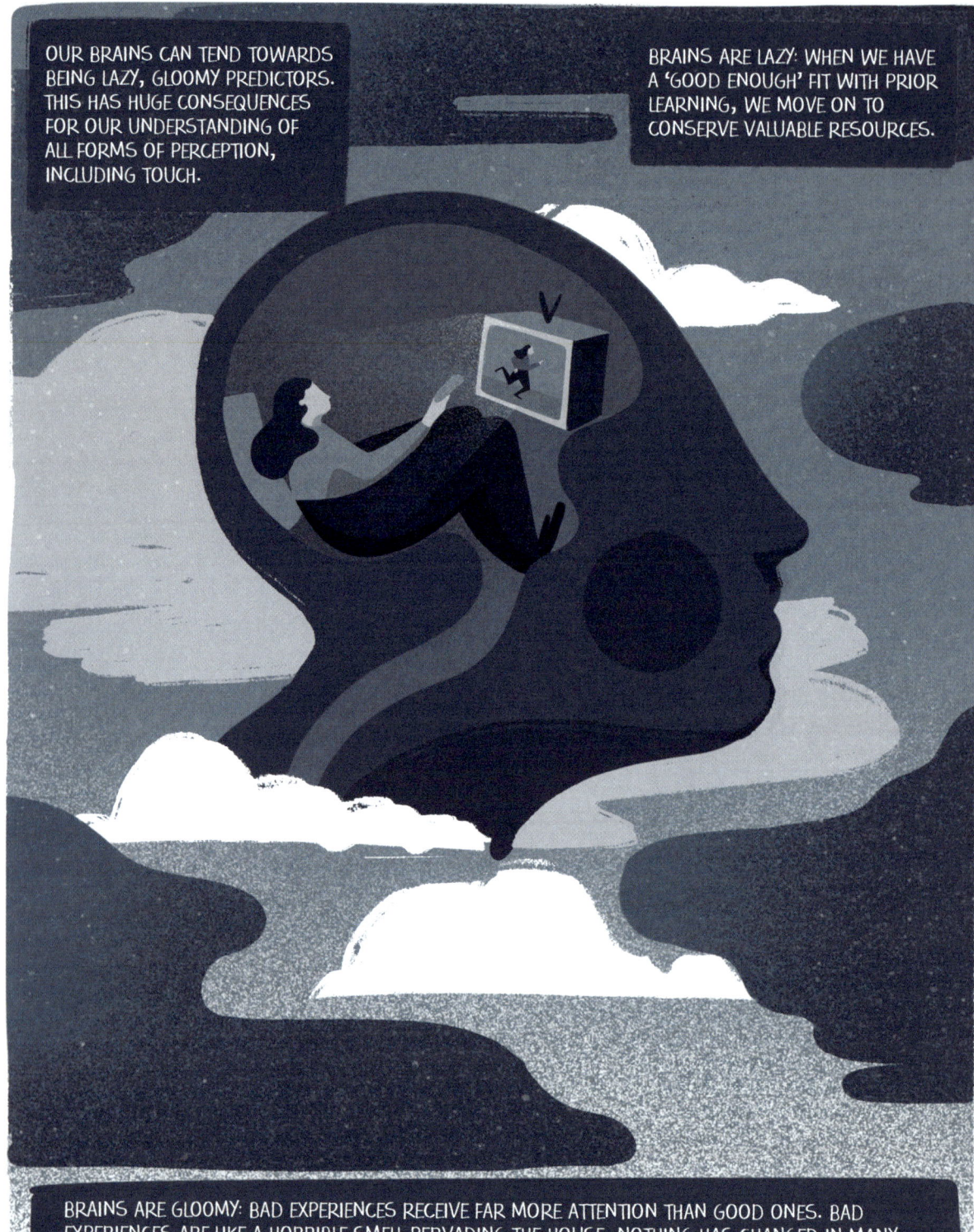

'It is essential to recognise that homeostasis drives behavior' (Craig 2015). 'The psychologist, Paul Rozin, an expert on disgust, observed that a single cockroach will completely wreck the appeal of a bowl of cherries, but a cherry will do nothing at all for a bowl of cockroaches' (Kahenman 2013).

'Your brain is predictive, not reactive.' 'Intrinsic brain activity is one of the great recent discoveries in neuroscience. Even more compelling is what this brain activity represents: millions of predictions of what you will encounter next in the world, based on your lifetime of past experience' (Barrett 2017).

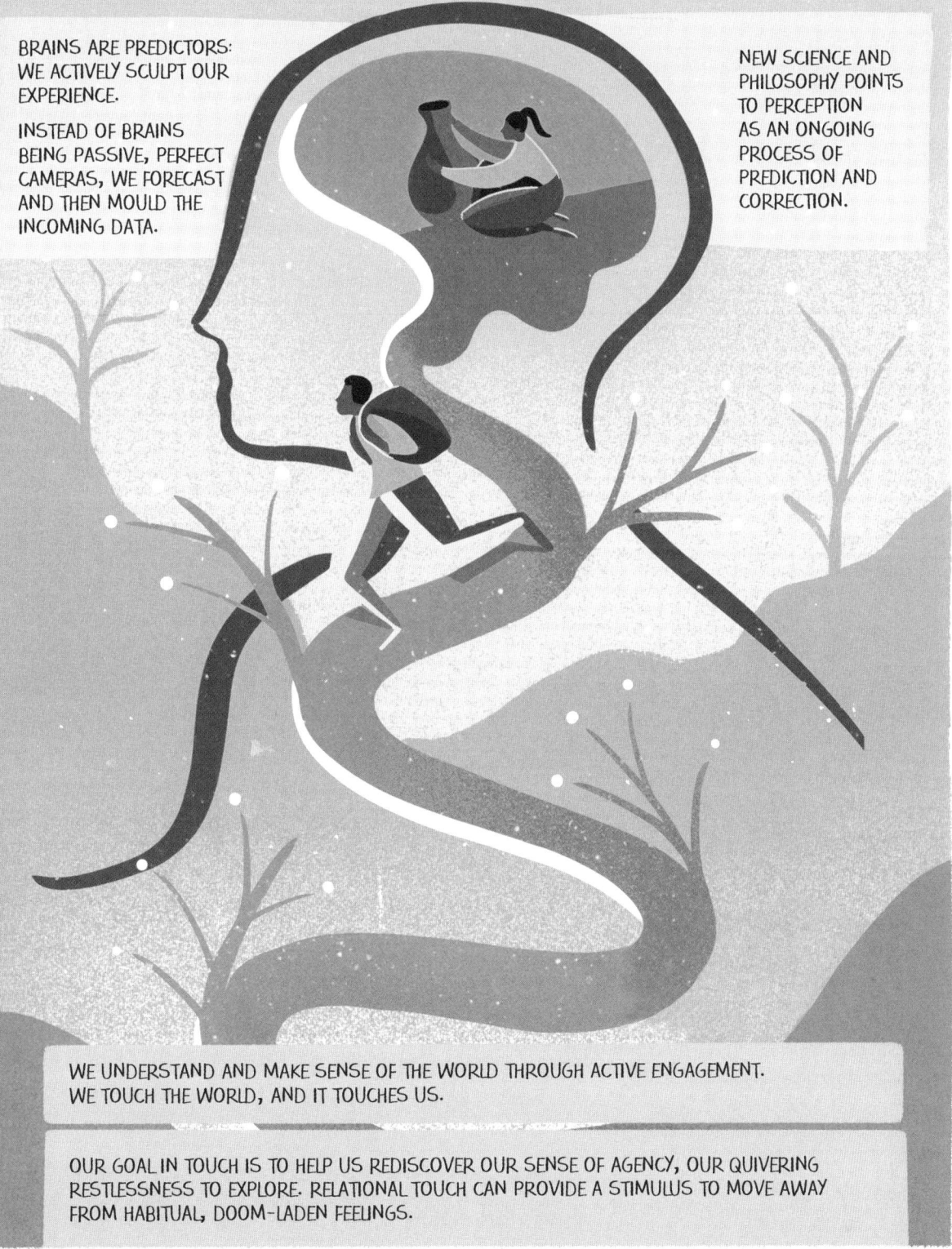

BRAINS ARE PREDICTORS: WE ACTIVELY SCULPT OUR EXPERIENCE.

INSTEAD OF BRAINS BEING PASSIVE, PERFECT CAMERAS, WE FORECAST AND THEN MOULD THE INCOMING DATA.

NEW SCIENCE AND PHILOSOPHY POINTS TO PERCEPTION AS AN ONGOING PROCESS OF PREDICTION AND CORRECTION.

WE UNDERSTAND AND MAKE SENSE OF THE WORLD THROUGH ACTIVE ENGAGEMENT. WE TOUCH THE WORLD, AND IT TOUCHES US.

OUR GOAL IN TOUCH IS TO HELP US REDISCOVER OUR SENSE OF AGENCY, OUR QUIVERING RESTLESSNESS TO EXPLORE. RELATIONAL TOUCH CAN PROVIDE A STIMULUS TO MOVE AWAY FROM HABITUAL, DOOM-LADEN FEELINGS.

'Unifying the senses depends on acting: doing, seeing and feeling, sensing the feedback from the doing at the same time' (Tversky 2019). The presence of another, amplified by safe touch, is a fantastic tool to help us interpret the feedback from the world and our bodies.

Aristotle on touch: 'its absence spells doom to man and all animals' (Courtney and Nolan 2017). The Libertines' song 'Can't Stand Me Now' summed up the sometimes overwhelming pushback: 'Cornered the boy kicked out at the world. The world kicked back a lot fuckin' harder now' (Doherty et al. 2004).

HOW DOES TOUCH WORK? FIRST, LET'S EXPAND OUR NOTION OF TOUCH.

TOUCH IS INEXTRICABLY LINKED WITH BODY AWARENESS. TOUCH IS USED HERE TO INCLUDE ANY SENSATIONS THAT HELP US FEEL.

IT WOULD BE A MISTAKE TO ISOLATE THE PERCEPTION OF TOUCH TO THINGS PRESSING AGAINST NERVES IN THE SKIN.

NERVES ARE NOT ONLY SENSITIVE AT THE RECEPTOR AT THE END OF THE NERVE. THERE ARE MEMBRANE CHANNELS ALONG THE WHOLE LENGTH OF THE NERVE THAT SOAK UP CHEMICAL SIGNALS SUCH AS STRESS HORMONES AND INFLAMMATORY MODULATORS.

WE ARE SUFFUSED WITH SENSORS. THEY TRACK CHANGES IN THE STATE OF TISSUES, CELL ACTIVITY AND THE FLUID CHEMICAL SOUP. AS IT TOUCHES THE WORLD, OUR PERCEPTION OF OUR BODY IS AFFECTED BY THE STATE OF THE OUTSIDE AND THE INSIDE OF THE BODY. WE TOUCH INWARD AS WELL AS OUTWARD.

TO MANAGE OUR SENSE OF TOUCH FURTHER, OUR BRAINS TURN UP OR TURN DOWN THE VOLUME OF SIGNALS THEY RECEIVE FROM OUR SENSORS, DEPENDING ON OUR GOALS AT THAT MOMENT.

Fulkerson (2020) describes models linking touch and interoception: 'The sense of touch is closely connected to bodily awareness.' '...many aspects of touch... are primarily directed not at the external world, but at the present state of our bodies.'

'Touch also enables us to sense the external environment, as well as has a role in shaping mental representations of our own body.' 'Bodily sensation is necessary for tactual perception' (Karasu 2020). Sensory neurons have extensive interactions with immune cells to create danger signals (Donnelly et al. 2020).

CLOSE YOUR EYES AND TRY TO TOUCH YOUR FINGER TO YOUR NOSE. YOU PROBABLY DIDN'T MISS BY TOO MUCH. THE SKILL TO MAP A MOVING BODY IN SPACE IS LARGELY POSSIBLE DUE TO QUICK SIGNALS: 'PROPRIOCEPTION' FROM MECHANORECEPTORS IN MUSCLES, LIGAMENTS AND JOINTS.

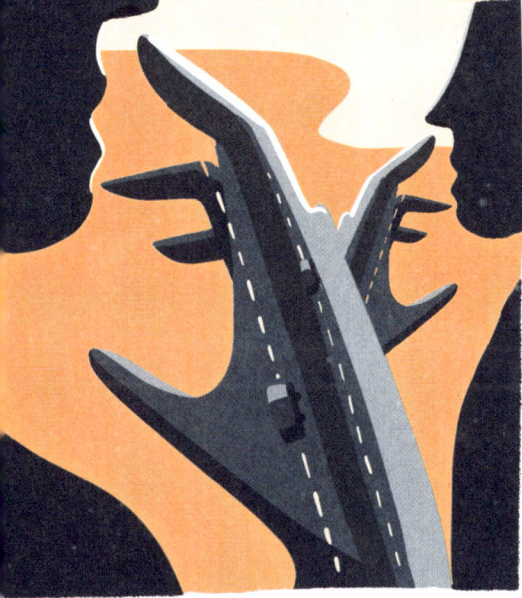

NOW CLOSE YOUR EYES AND HOLD YOUR ARM IN THE AIR. HOW DO YOU KNOW YOU HAVE AN ARM? TUNE INTO THE TEMPERATURE, THE WEIGHT, THE ITCH, THE FLOW INSIDE – FIND THE ESSENTIAL 'ARMNESS' OF AN ARM.

THIS IS LARGELY SLOW SIGNALS, 'INTEROCEPTION' FROM FREE NERVE ENDINGS.

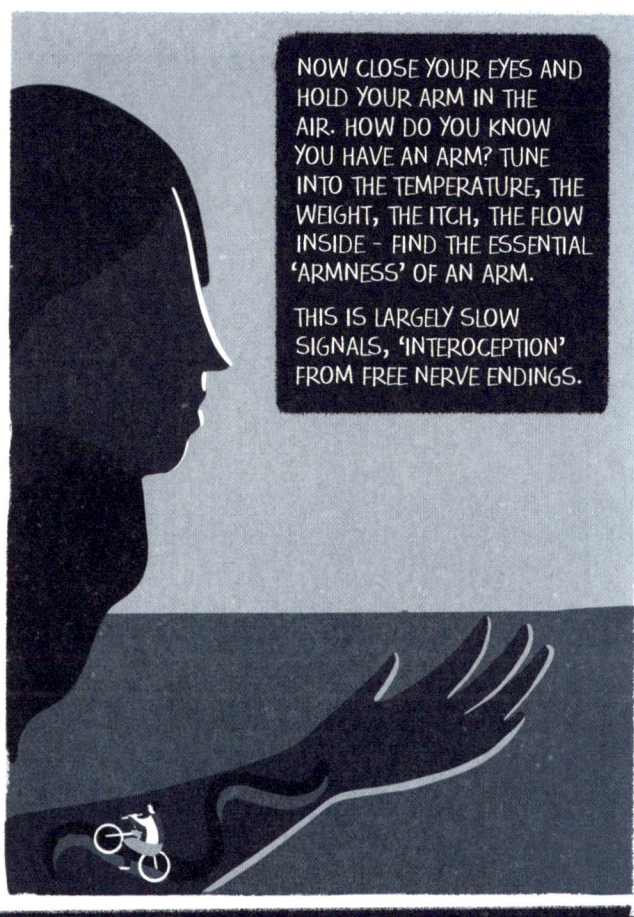

IT IS USEFUL TO DISTINGUISH TWO TYPES OF TOUCH – SLOW TOUCH AND QUICK TOUCH. QUICK TOUCH GOES ALONG BIG, INSULATED (MYELINATED), FAST NERVES (A-FIBRES). THINK OF THEM AS MOTORWAYS TRANSPORTING LOTS OF MOVEMENT SIGNALS.

SLOW TOUCH GOES ALONG SMALL, UNINSULATED, SLOW NERVES (C-FIBRES). THINK OF THEM AS SMALL COUNTRY LANES AND PATHS.

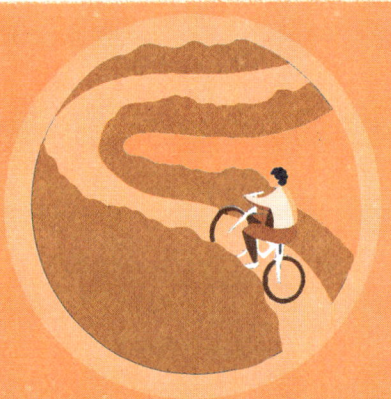

IT TURNS OUT OUR COUNTRY LANES AND PATHS CARRY THE VAST MAJORITY OF SIGNALS TO THE BRAIN. THEY ARE CENTRAL TO FEELING AND CONSCIOUSNESS, TRANSPORTING THE ESSENTIAL STUFF OF EXISTENCE.

'Only 25% of somatosensory afferent nerves are in fact A-fibers, with unmyelinated C-fibers constituting the majority of afferents in all mammalian species.' C-fibres are '50 times slower' and carry gentle touch, 'providing the neurobiological sub-strate for the development and function of the social brain' (McGlone et al. 2014).

Interoception is the slow background tone of the body. 'Interoception can be trained' (Craig 2015). This book is framing interoception as 'inward touch'. The 'felt sense' is a wonderful term from the focusing tradition that celebrates the distinct quality of inward touch that meets the core, hidden, emotional stories in our bodies (Gendlin 1981).

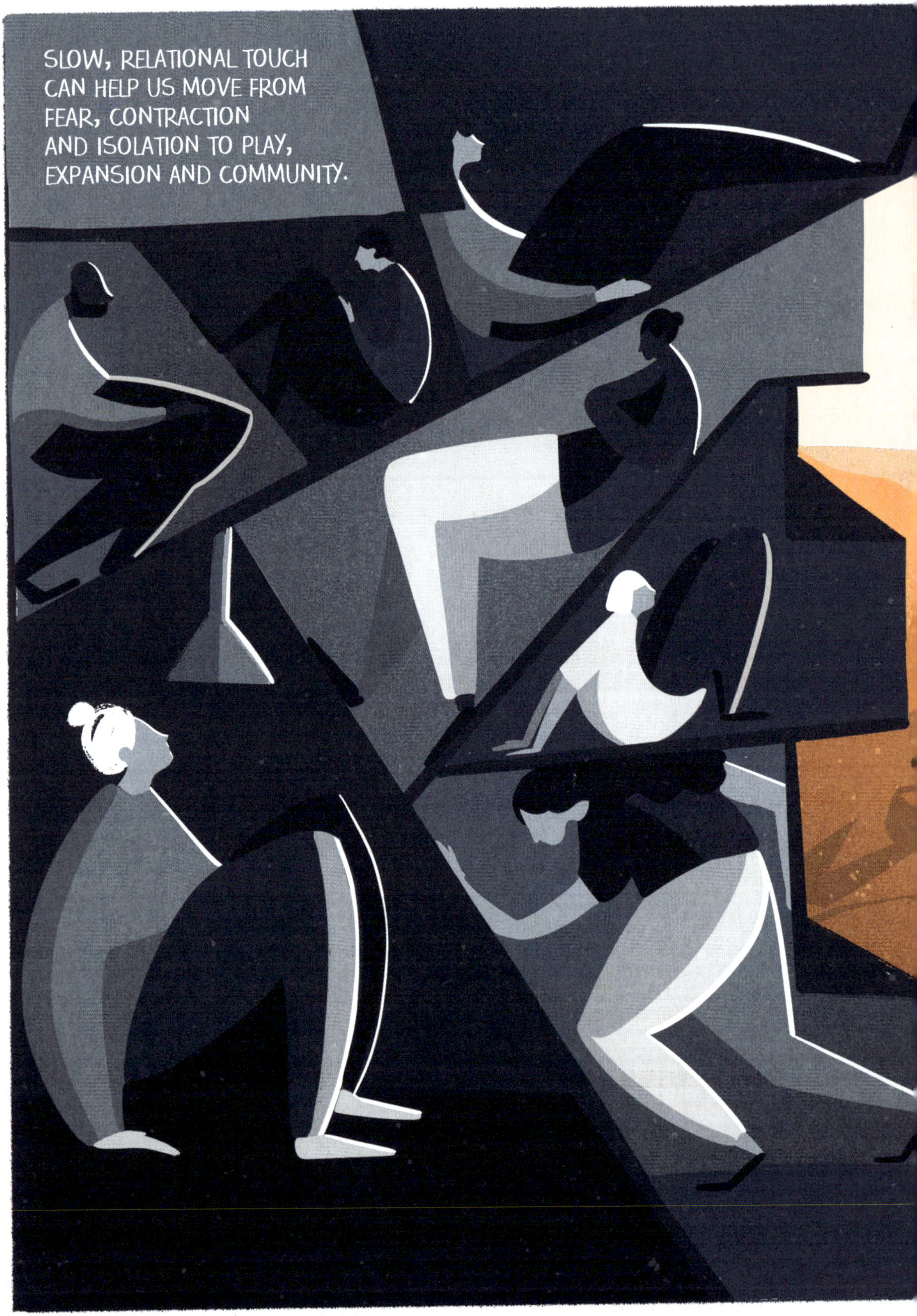
SLOW, RELATIONAL TOUCH CAN HELP US MOVE FROM FEAR, CONTRACTION AND ISOLATION TO PLAY, EXPANSION AND COMMUNITY.

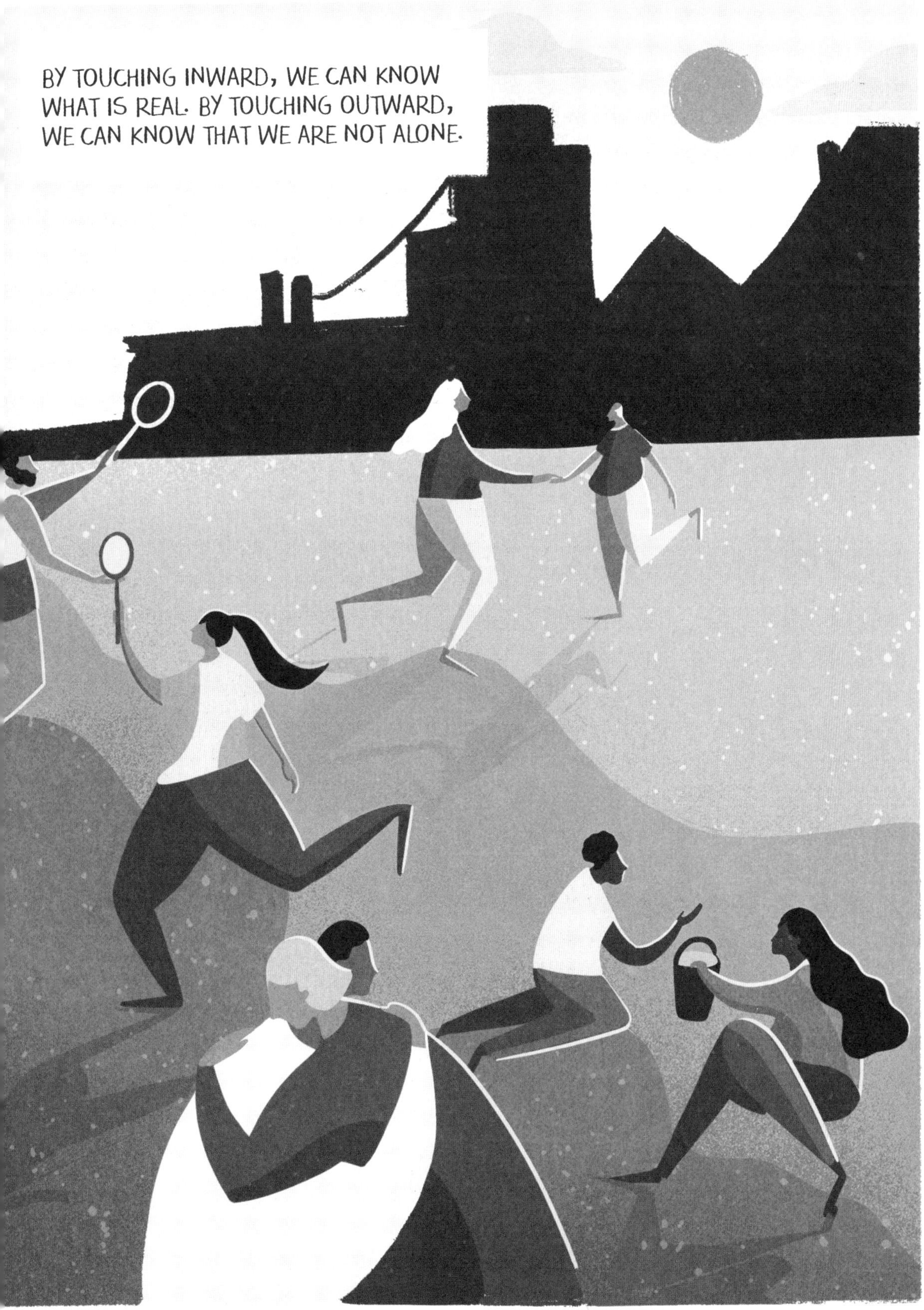
BY TOUCHING INWARD, WE CAN KNOW WHAT IS REAL. BY TOUCHING OUTWARD, WE CAN KNOW THAT WE ARE NOT ALONE.

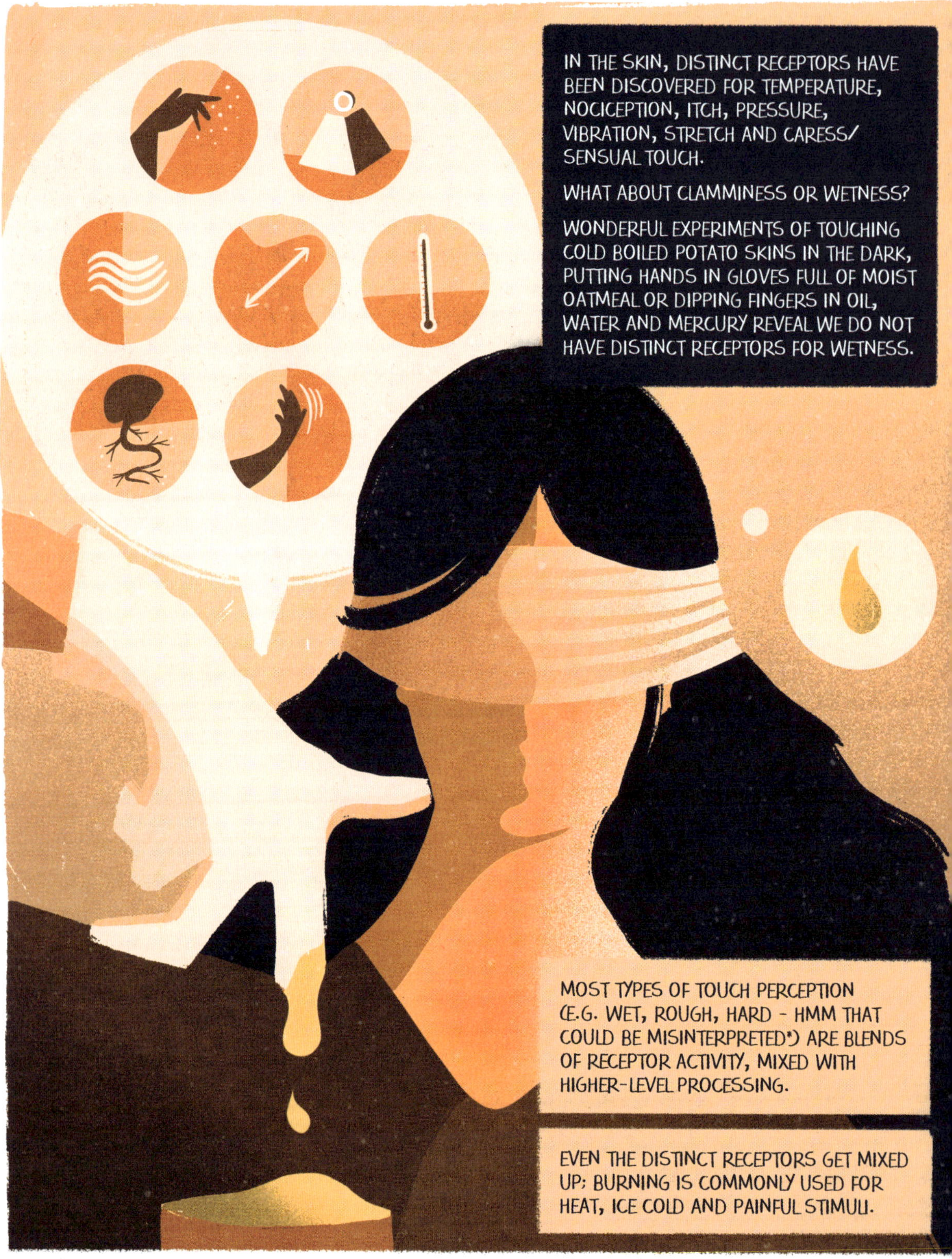
IN THE SKIN, DISTINCT RECEPTORS HAVE BEEN DISCOVERED FOR TEMPERATURE, NOCICEPTION, ITCH, PRESSURE, VIBRATION, STRETCH AND CARESS/ SENSUAL TOUCH.
WHAT ABOUT CLAMMINESS OR WETNESS?
WONDERFUL EXPERIMENTS OF TOUCHING COLD BOILED POTATO SKINS IN THE DARK, PUTTING HANDS IN GLOVES FULL OF MOIST OATMEAL OR DIPPING FINGERS IN OIL, WATER AND MERCURY REVEAL WE DO NOT HAVE DISTINCT RECEPTORS FOR WETNESS.
MOST TYPES OF TOUCH PERCEPTION (E.G. WET, ROUGH, HARD - HMM THAT COULD BE MISINTERPRETED*) ARE BLENDS OF RECEPTOR ACTIVITY, MIXED WITH HIGHER-LEVEL PROCESSING.
EVEN THE DISTINCT RECEPTORS GET MIXED UP; BURNING IS COMMONLY USED FOR HEAT, ICE COLD AND PAINFUL STIMULI.

We respond to thermal, chemical and physical stimuli. The epidermis (the outer skin layer) and the dermis and superficial fascia underneath contain lots of nerves. *Unfortunately this book does not cover erotic touch, it's different... However, see Parkinson (2020) for a nice riff on erotic touch.

We do not have pain receptors. Nociceptors are 'danger receptors' for a stimulus that is too much or too quick. That nociceptors are danger receptors and not pain receptors is a canonical belief in the Explain Pain paradigm (Moseley and Butler 2017). For touch experiments (and a chapter on sexual touch) see Linden (2015).

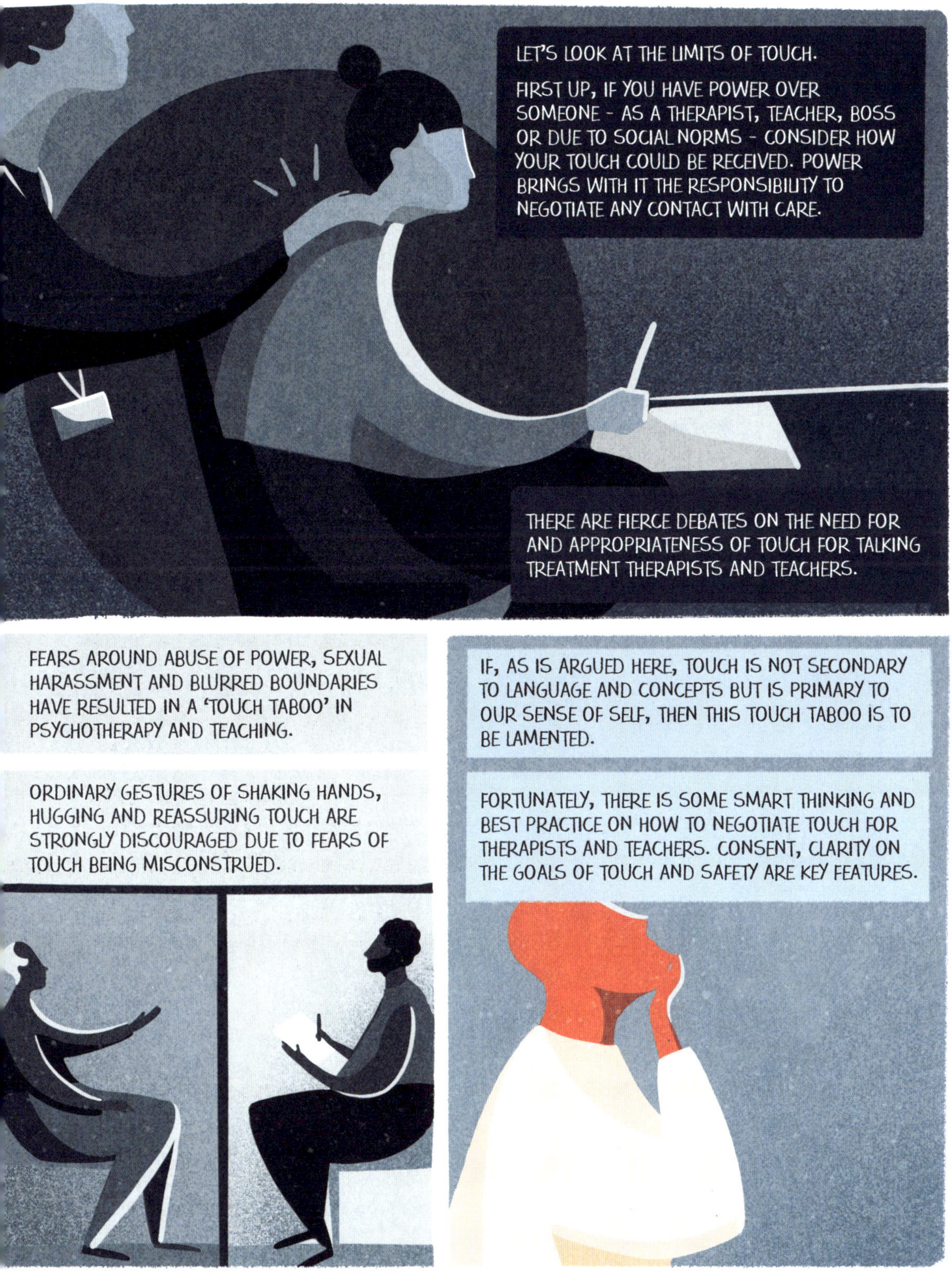
LET'S LOOK AT THE LIMITS OF TOUCH.
FIRST UP, IF YOU HAVE POWER OVER SOMEONE - AS A THERAPIST, TEACHER, BOSS OR DUE TO SOCIAL NORMS - CONSIDER HOW YOUR TOUCH COULD BE RECEIVED. POWER BRINGS WITH IT THE RESPONSIBILITY TO NEGOTIATE ANY CONTACT WITH CARE.
THERE ARE FIERCE DEBATES ON THE NEED FOR AND APPROPRIATENESS OF TOUCH FOR TALKING TREATMENT THERAPISTS AND TEACHERS.
FEARS AROUND ABUSE OF POWER, SEXUAL HARASSMENT AND BLURRED BOUNDARIES HAVE RESULTED IN A 'TOUCH TABOO' IN PSYCHOTHERAPY AND TEACHING.
ORDINARY GESTURES OF SHAKING HANDS, HUGGING AND REASSURING TOUCH ARE STRONGLY DISCOURAGED DUE TO FEARS OF TOUCH BEING MISCONSTRUED.
IF, AS IS ARGUED HERE, TOUCH IS NOT SECONDARY TO LANGUAGE AND CONCEPTS BUT IS PRIMARY TO OUR SENSE OF SELF, THEN THIS TOUCH TABOO IS TO BE LAMENTED.
FORTUNATELY, THERE IS SOME SMART THINKING AND BEST PRACTICE ON HOW TO NEGOTIATE TOUCH FOR THERAPISTS AND TEACHERS. CONSENT, CLARITY ON THE GOALS OF TOUCH AND SAFETY ARE KEY FEATURES.

'In spite of the numerous therapeutic approaches...that systematically and effectively use touch in therapy, touch has nevertheless been marginalized, forbidden, called a taboo, often sexualized, and at times, even criminalized by many schools of psychotherapy and ethicists' (Zur and Nordmarken 2020).

'Several factors have been found to significantly correlate with a client's positive evaluation of touch, such as clarity regarding boundaries, congruence of touch, client's sense of being in control and the client's perception that touch is for his/her benefit' (Zur and Nordmarken 2020).

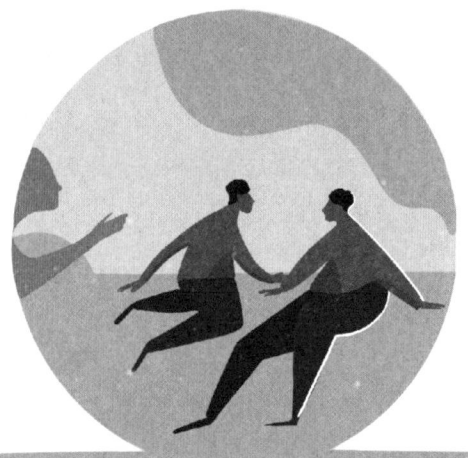

WE NEED TO BE SENSITIVE TO CULTURAL NORMS. AMERICAN ADOLESCENTS TOUCHED EACH OTHER LESS AND WERE MORE AGGRESSIVE COMPARED TO FRENCH ADOLESCENTS WHEN OBSERVED IN PUBLIC.

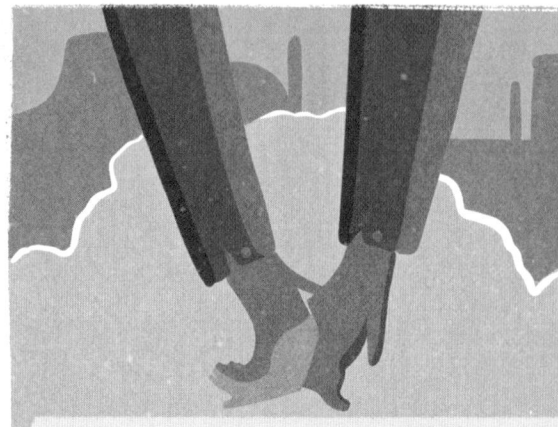

MEN HOLDING HANDS? DEEPLY NORMAL IN MANY PARTS OF THE MIDDLE EAST AND AFRICA. DEEPLY STRANGE IN NORTH AMERICA AND MANY PARTS OF EUROPE.

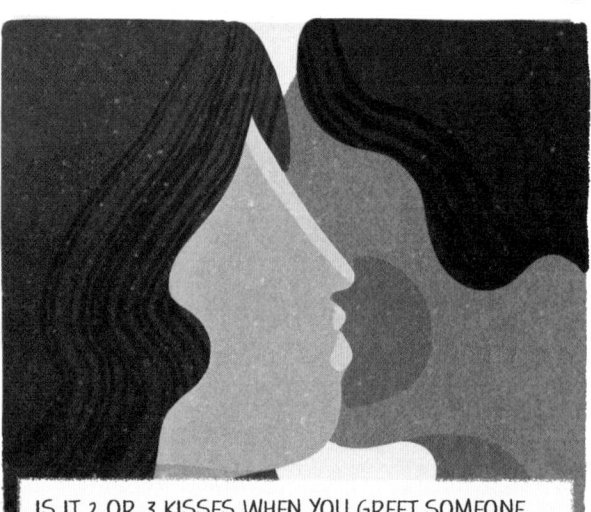

IS IT 2 OR 3 KISSES WHEN YOU GREET SOMEONE IN PARTS OF EUROPE? SHOULD WE ALL LEARN TO NAMASTE, A NON-CONTACT GREETING FROM INDIA?

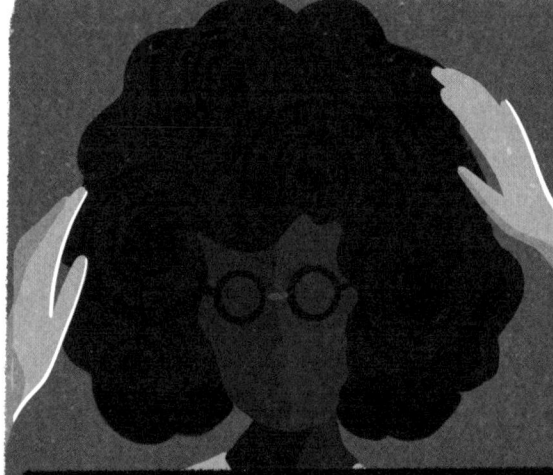

WE CAN ALSO EXPRESS UNCONSCIOUS RACISM THROUGH TOUCH. 'CAN I TOUCH YOUR HAIR?' IS A MICROAGGRESSION AND RARELY ACCEPTABLE FOR A WHITE PERSON TO ASK A BLACK PERSON.

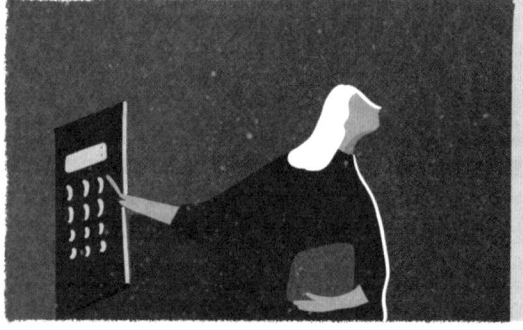

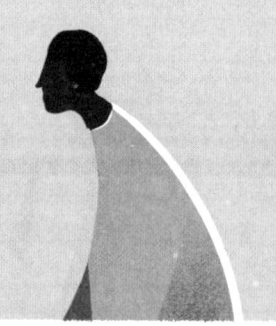

NOT BEING PREPARED TO TOUCH SOMEONE OR MOVING AWAY FROM SOMEONE, FOR EXAMPLE IN AN ELEVATOR, BECAUSE OF THEIR RACE IS A MICROAGGRESSION.

A classic 1966 study by S Jourard counted how many times two people touched in cafés around the world: London 0, Florida 2, Paris 110, Puerto Rico 180. Field, in her own research in 1999, found similar results observing teens in McDonalds in Paris and Miami (Field 2001).

'OMG. Can I touch your hair? Yeah that drove me mad.' A young mixed race woman powerfully describes acts of racism growing up in south of England (Gordon 2020). For a skit 'Racism in the elevator', see Reckless Tortuga (2008).

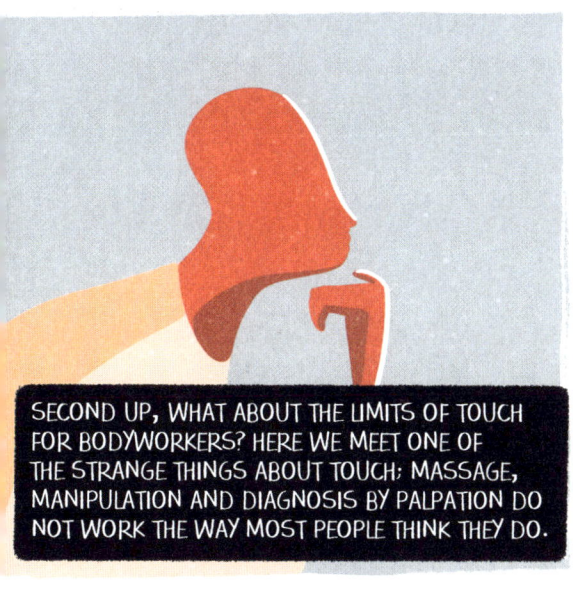

THE CLASSIC MODEL IS THAT MASSAGE WORKS BY POKING, PRODDING, RUBBING, MANIPULATING OR STRETCHING INDIVIDUAL PARTS OF THE BODY.

TOUCH THERAPISTS OFTEN AIM TO BREAK DOWN SCAR TISSUE OR MASSAGE OUT KNOTS OR ALIGN JOINTS OR ACCURATELY DIAGNOSE BY TOUCH.

SECOND UP, WHAT ABOUT THE LIMITS OF TOUCH FOR BODYWORKERS? HERE WE MEET ONE OF THE STRANGE THINGS ABOUT TOUCH; MASSAGE, MANIPULATION AND DIAGNOSIS BY PALPATION DO NOT WORK THE WAY MOST PEOPLE THINK THEY DO.

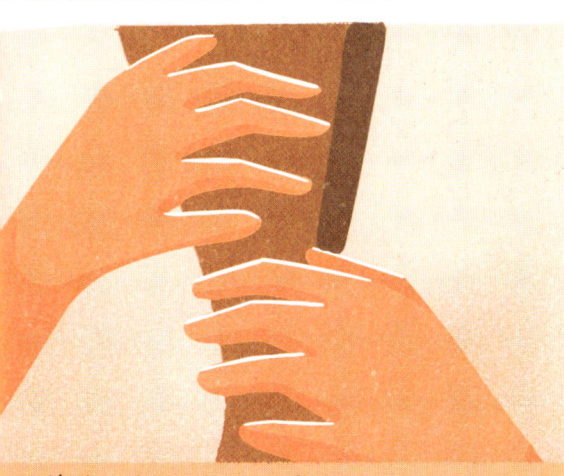

IF YOUR ANKLE HURTS, LET'S TOUCH THE ANKLE TO FIX THE ANKLE. THE THERAPIST WILL DIRECT INTERVENTIONS TO AFFECT THE STATE OF THE LOCAL TISSUES - FASCIA, MUSCLES, LIGAMENTS, SKIN OR JOINTS.

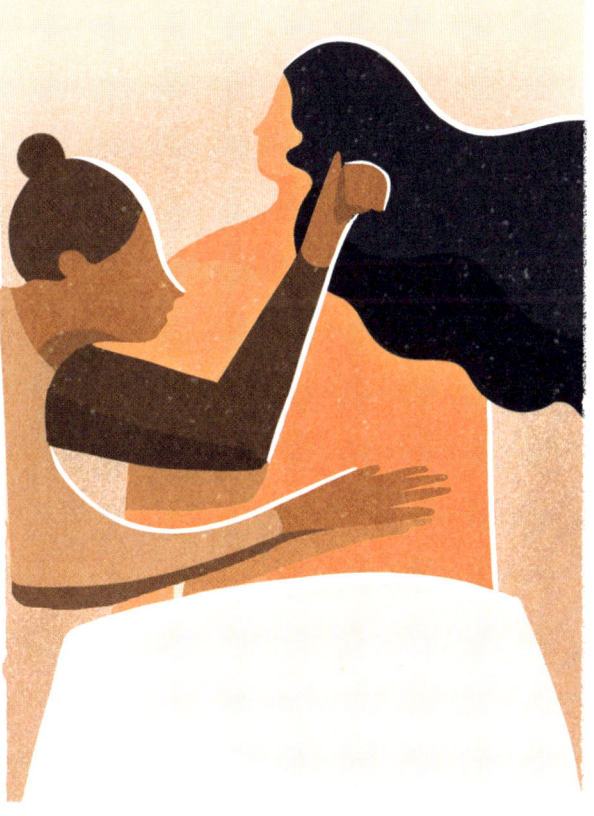

UNFORTUNATELY, THERE IS VERY LITTLE EVIDENCE THAT THIS FRAMEWORK OF DIRECT INTERVENTIONS PROVIDES ANY LASTING, MEANINGFUL CHANGE.

TIME TO PUT AWAY YOUR FOAM ROLLERS AND RE-THINK STICKING ELBOWS INTO MUSCLES... YOU DON'T NEED TO GIVE PAIN TO CHANGE PAIN.

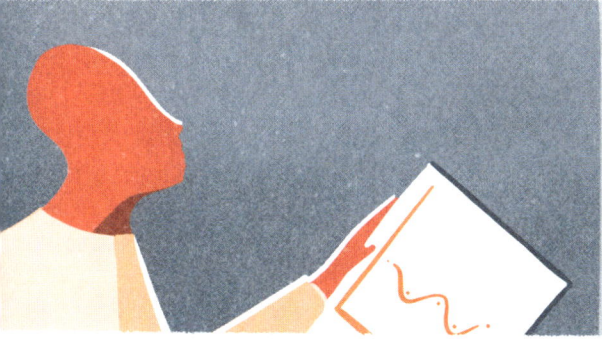

Pain, inflammation and the defence cascades of trauma are protective reflexes. The link that triggers all these outputs to protect is the perception of danger. 'To reduce pain, we need to reduce credible evidence of danger and increase credible evidence of safety' (Moseley and Butler 2017).

Best practice is now seen as listening to the patient, diagnosing biopsychosocial factors, explaining pain science and encouraging moving without fear to load tissues. Use touch and movement to offer 'nice, novel, safe input into the neuro-immune representation in the brain' (Butler 2015).

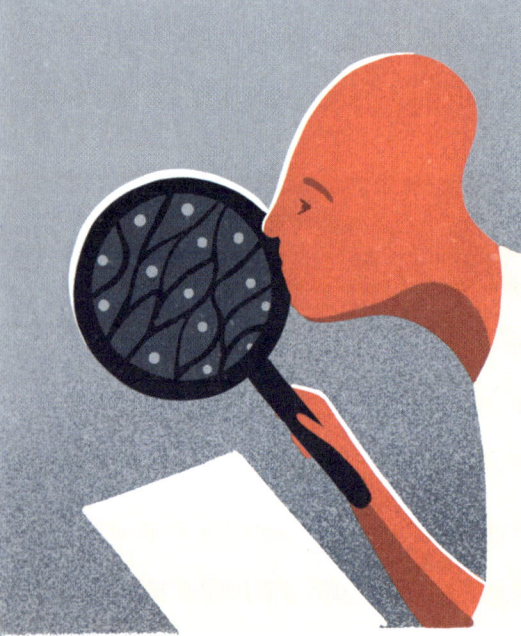

WE CAN'T RELIABLY DIAGNOSE BY TOUCH.

'INTER-OPERATOR RELIABILITY', WHERE EXPERTS COMPARE THEIR DIAGNOSIS OF, SAY, THE POSITION OF A SCAPULA OR THE TENSION IN A MUSCLE, IS VERY POOR IN MANUAL THERAPY.

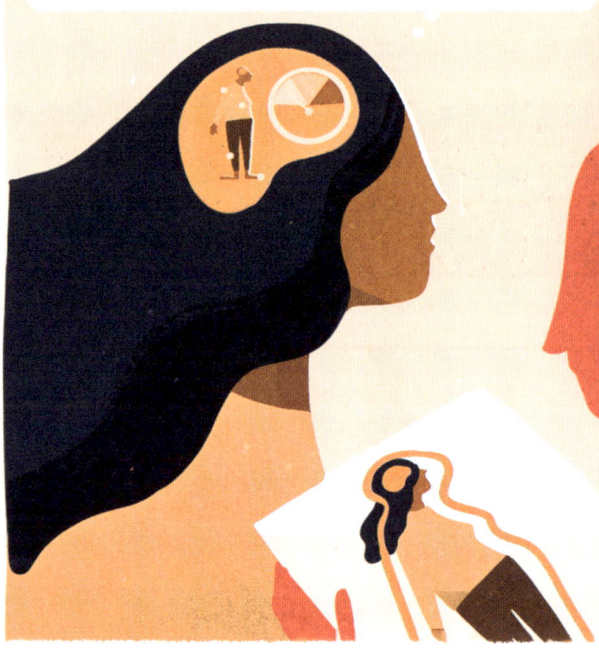

WE CAN'T CHANGE TISSUES BY PRIMARILY LOCALLY FOCUSED TOUCH.

TISSUES CHANGE BECAUSE THE PERSON CHANGES. THE REPRESENTATION IN THE BRAIN, NOT LOCAL TISSUES, SHOULD BE THE FOCUS FOR MANUAL THERAPISTS. THE REPRESENTATION IS ENTIRELY DEPENDENT ON THE PERCEPTION OF SAFETY.

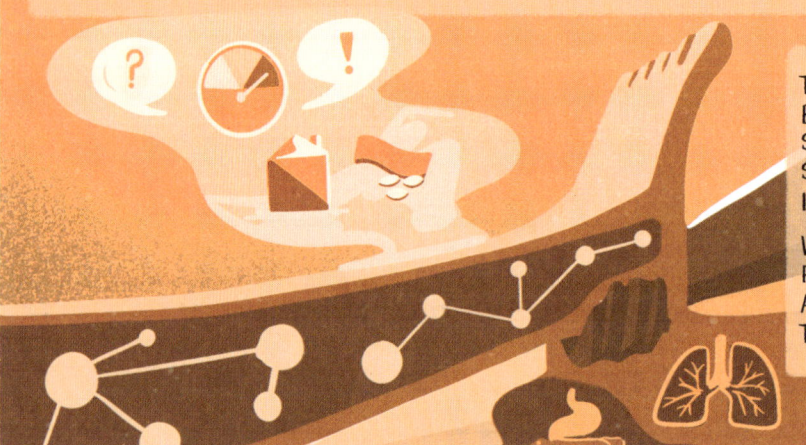

EVEN IF WE COULD DIAGNOSE AND THEN CHANGE TISSUES, IT DOESN'T REALLY MATTER.

THERE IS A TSUNAMI OF EVIDENCE THAT BETTER BIOMECHANICS, HOWEVER DEFINED, DOES NOT CONSISTENTLY LEAD TO LESS PAIN.

THE GOAL OF TOUCH SHOULD NOT BE LOCAL DYNAMICS. THE GOAL SHOULD BE A SAFE, MEANINGFUL STIMULUS TO ENGAGE A PERSON IN THEIR WORLD.

WE TOUCH WHOLE PEOPLE, NOT PARTS OF PEOPLE. ALWAYS. ACKNOWLEDGE THAT AND IT IS TRANSFORMATIVE.

'Many "biomechanical" variables can't be reliably assessed and/or don't correlate with pain.' 'Injury doesn't always equal pain. Psychosocial factors can play a huge role in pain' (Bowman 2017). There is an existential crisis in physiotherapy as research constantly dismantles some of the sacred cows of manual therapy.

'In the slow transition away from manual therapy we are seeing a shift in the practice of our profession, where the abandonment of hands on approaches in patient care is being applauded by some...and some of our educational institutions are debating if we should even educate physical therapy students to mobilize and manipulate' (MacDonald et al. 2020).

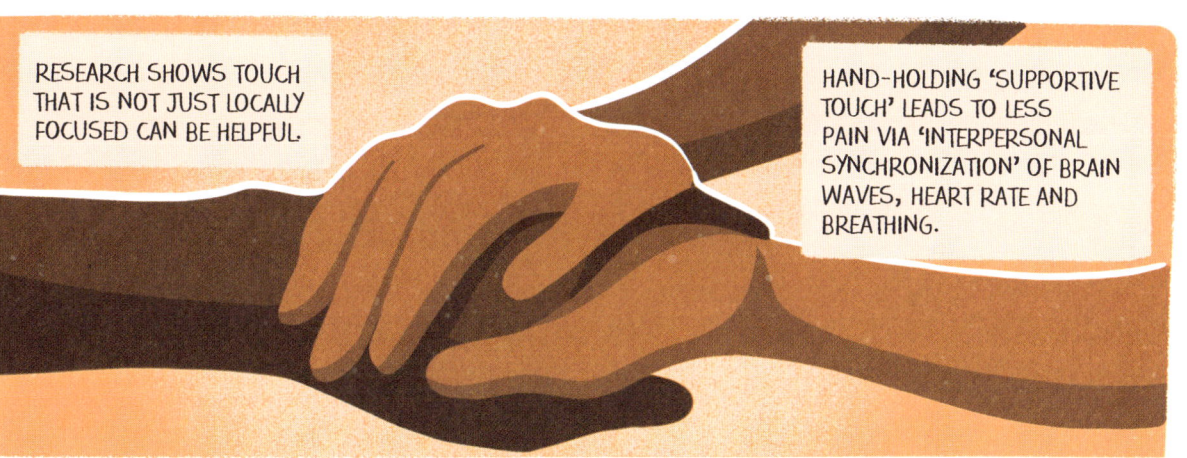

RESEARCH SHOWS TOUCH THAT IS NOT JUST LOCALLY FOCUSED CAN BE HELPFUL.

HAND-HOLDING 'SUPPORTIVE TOUCH' LEADS TO LESS PAIN VIA 'INTERPERSONAL SYNCHRONIZATION' OF BRAIN WAVES, HEART RATE AND BREATHING.

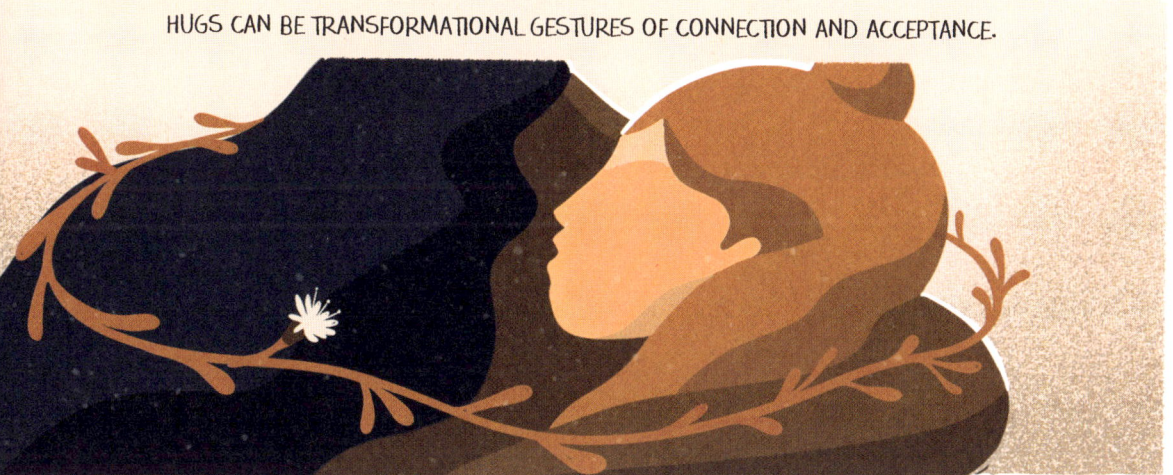

HUGS CAN BE TRANSFORMATIONAL GESTURES OF CONNECTION AND ACCEPTANCE.

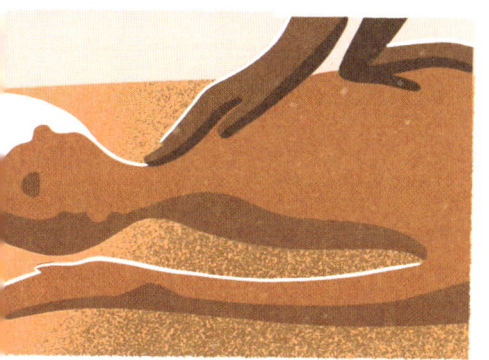

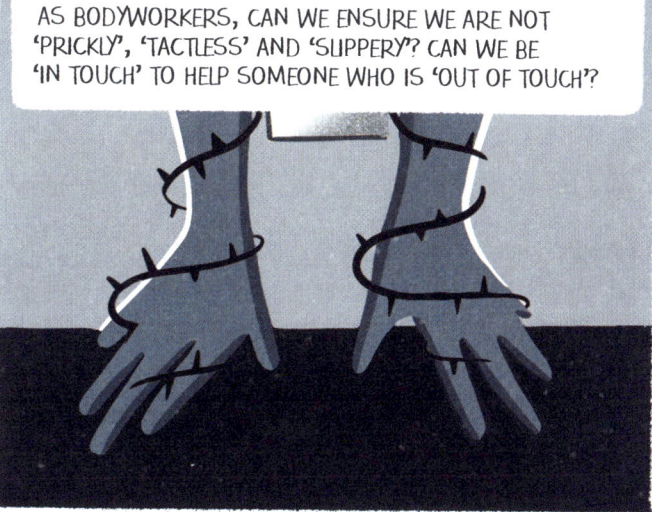

AS BODYWORKERS, CAN WE ENSURE WE ARE NOT 'PRICKLY', 'TACTLESS' AND 'SLIPPERY'? CAN WE BE 'IN TOUCH' TO HELP SOMEONE WHO IS 'OUT OF TOUCH'?

PROFESSOR TIFFANY FIELD, A VERY INFLUENTIAL FIGURE IN TOUCH, FOUND 'MASSAGE THERAPY HAS SIGNIFICANTLY REDUCED PAIN AND INCREASED FUNCTION IN ALL OF THE CHRONIC PAIN SYNDROME STUDIES THAT HAVE BEEN PUBLISHED OVER THE LAST DECADE.'

'Touch is an exquisitely social sense, capable of allowing accurate communication of specific emotional states. Interpersonal touch is associated with wellbeing, promoting pleasant feelings, approach-related behaviors, and reductions in aversive feelings and acute pain' (López-Solà et al. 2019). Field (2018), quoted above, reviewed pain and massage research.

'Free Mom Hugs' and 'Free Dad Hugs' at LGBTQ events in the US are wonderful examples of the simple power of a hug. 'Being a trauma-informed bodyworker is like learning a new language' (Olson 2020). 'Pain science matters as a component of comprehensive patient management and clinical reasoning, but not to replace hands-on approaches' (MacDonald et al. 2020).

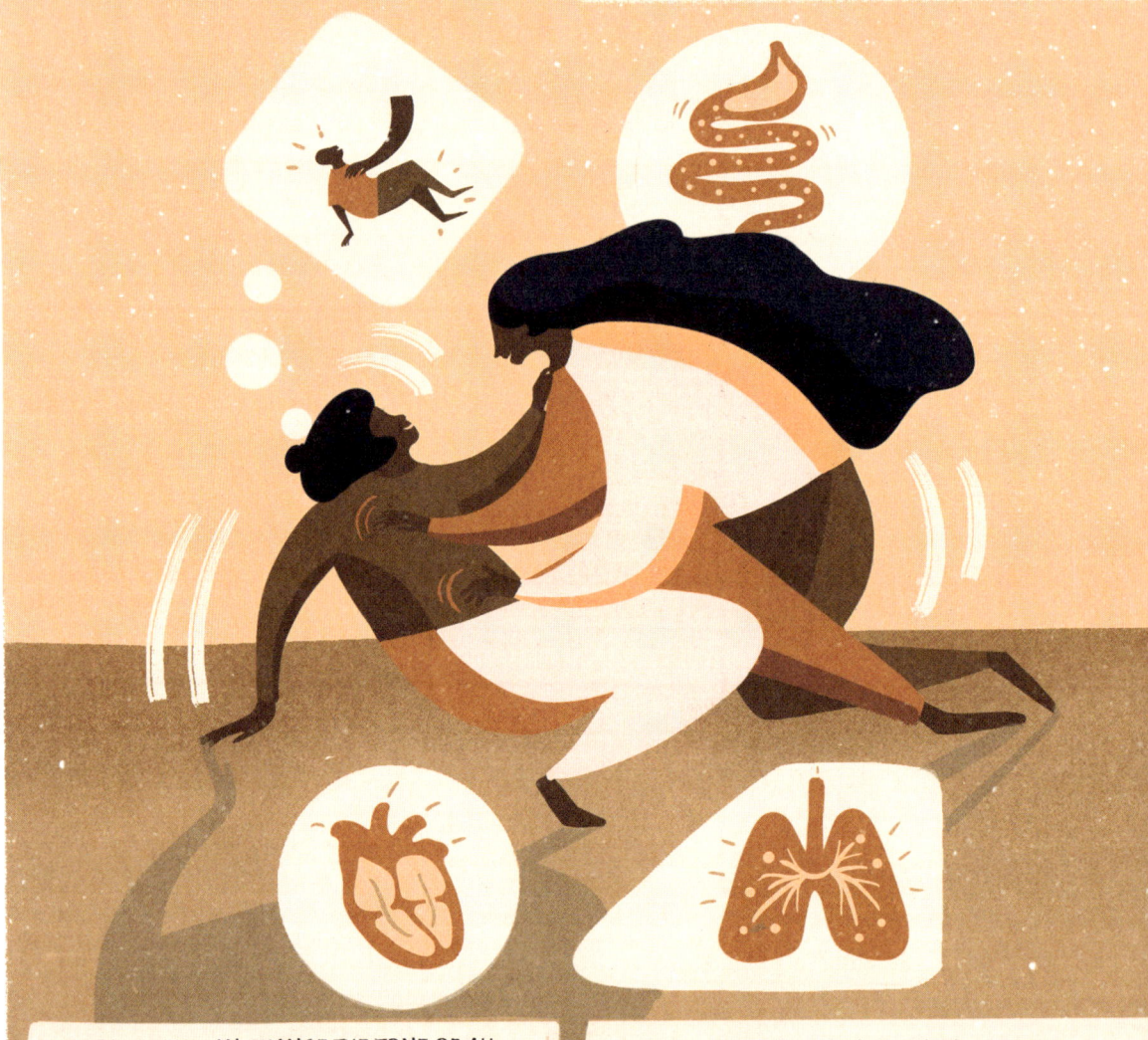

SO, HAVING MADE A CASE FOR THE NEED FOR TOUCH AND ACKNOWLEDGED THE LIMITS OF TOUCH, HOW CAN WE DEVELOP OUR TOUCH SKILLS?

LET'S THINK ABOUT BEING TICKLED.

A TINY STIMULUS CAN CHANGE EVERY SYSTEM IN OUR BODIES AND GENERATE A HOST OF MEMORIES AND EMOTIONS.

THE BEAUTY OF TICKLING IS THAT IT IS A MIX OF SAFETY AND DANGER. IT IS INHERENTLY RELATIONAL. WE CANNOT TICKLE OURSELVES – IT'S NEVER QUITE SCARY ENOUGH.

A GOOD TICKLE CAN CHANGE THE TONE OF ALL YOUR MUSCLES, SHIFT YOUR BREATHING, CHANGE YOUR HEART RATE, ALMOST CERTAINLY REDUCE YOUR GUT ACTIVITY AND CHANGE YOUR HORMONE SECRETIONS. TO DEFEND THE TICKLE, YOU WILL SWITCH TO SHORT-TERM DEFENCE STRATEGIES.

IT IS TO BE HOPED THAT YOUR MEMORIES OF TICKLING ARE PLEASANT. SOME PEOPLE HATE IT – TOO MANY BAD MEMORIES OF FEELING HELPLESS AND OVERWHELMED, EVEN IF THE INTENTION WAS FUN.

IT'S A COMPLEX RESPONSE TO A SMALL STIMULUS.

'Most people can't tickle themselves effectively; the tactile sensation from self-tickling is much weaker than that which results from being tickled by another' (Linden 2015). Relational touch is a novel term, rooted in Taoist and Zen notions of 'less is more' and non-doing. It is often light, still-hands touch, but can include brushing or strong, deep, rhythmic touch.

The intention when touching is of fundamental importance. Relational touch is always about connecting to the whole person and all the stories they hold. 'Supportive touch', defined as 'interpersonal touch with an intention of providing emotional support', is a similar framework (López-Solà et al. 2019).

RELATIONAL TOUCH CAN BE DEFINED AS NON-DOING TOUCH THAT MEETS THE WHOLE PERSON. THE POWER OF RELATIONAL TOUCH CAN BE EASILY UNDERSTOOD BY APPRECIATING WHAT HAPPENS IN A TICKLE.

TOUCH IS AN INTIMATE ACT OF COMMUNICATION. TOUCH CAN RECONNECT US TO EARLY EXPERIENCES OF NEGOTIATING SAFETY AND AGENCY.

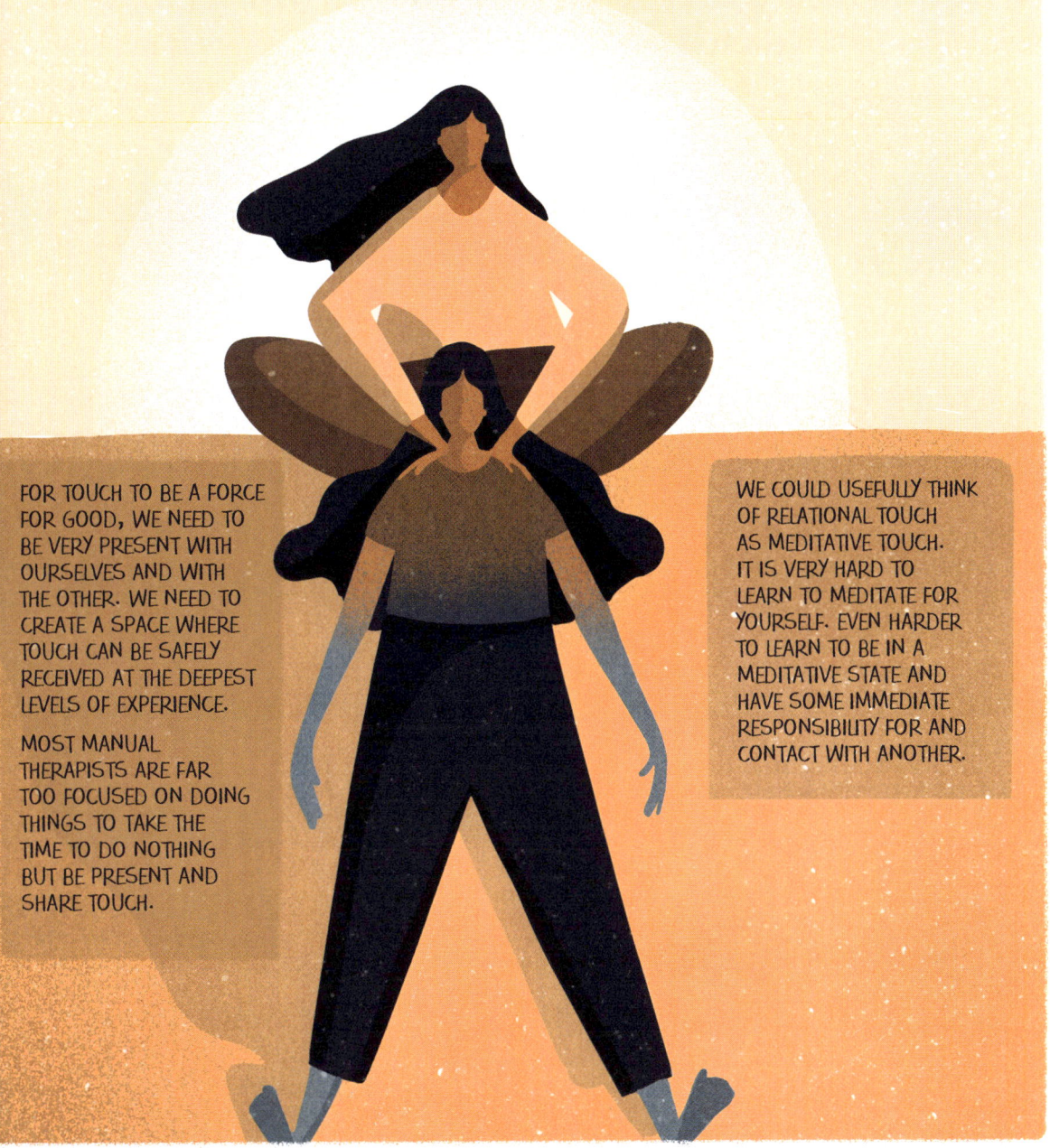

FOR TOUCH TO BE A FORCE FOR GOOD, WE NEED TO BE VERY PRESENT WITH OURSELVES AND WITH THE OTHER. WE NEED TO CREATE A SPACE WHERE TOUCH CAN BE SAFELY RECEIVED AT THE DEEPEST LEVELS OF EXPERIENCE.

MOST MANUAL THERAPISTS ARE FAR TOO FOCUSED ON DOING THINGS TO TAKE THE TIME TO DO NOTHING BUT BE PRESENT AND SHARE TOUCH.

WE COULD USEFULLY THINK OF RELATIONAL TOUCH AS MEDITATIVE TOUCH. IT IS VERY HARD TO LEARN TO MEDITATE FOR YOURSELF. EVEN HARDER TO LEARN TO BE IN A MEDITATIVE STATE AND HAVE SOME IMMEDIATE RESPONSIBILITY FOR AND CONTACT WITH ANOTHER.

I come from a tradition – biodynamic craniosacral therapy (BCST) – where still-hands touch and a huge focus on being present and safe are the core treatment skills. Like most manual therapies, the profession needs to do some philosophical housekeeping. Some of the core tenets, based on ropey biomechanics on one hand and unprovable mystic statements on the other, can easily be let go of.

A deep understanding within BCST that there is trauma and a need for embodied safety, that early experience leaves a trail in the flesh, that humans are polyrhythmic, and that those rhythms are information rich and influenced by skilful touch, still leaves a very exciting modality.
BCST, at its best, is a profound practice of non-doing relational touch.

TRY SOMETHING NOW.

TOUCH EXERCISE NO 1: SHIFTING PERCEPTION.

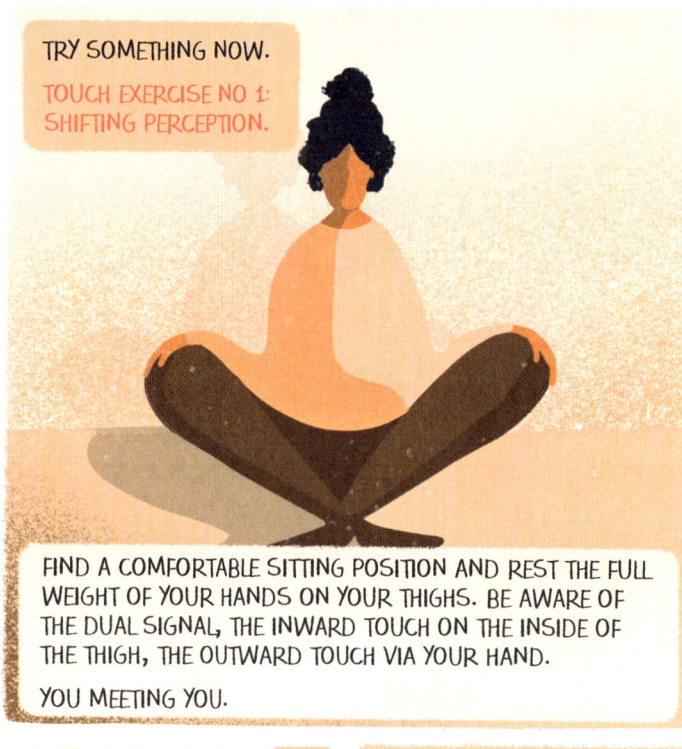

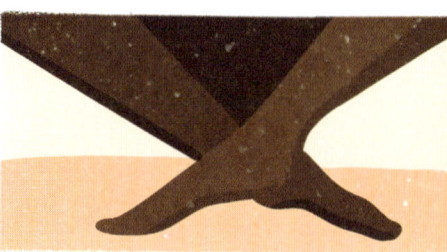

WHAT DO YOU NOTICE? MAYBE YOU CAN FEEL THE TONE OF YOUR MUSCLES, MAYBE FLOWING BLOOD, MAYBE A SENSE OF THE BONE DEEP IN THE MIDDLE. HOW DOES THE RIGHT COMPARE TO THE LEFT? THEY ARE RARELY THE SAME.

FIND A COMFORTABLE SITTING POSITION AND REST THE FULL WEIGHT OF YOUR HANDS ON YOUR THIGHS. BE AWARE OF THE DUAL SIGNAL, THE INWARD TOUCH ON THE INSIDE OF THE THIGH, THE OUTWARD TOUCH VIA YOUR HAND.

YOU MEETING YOU.

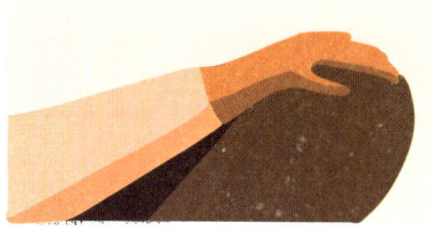

NOW LET'S TRY A PERCEPTUAL TRICK. KEEP CONTACT BUT MAKE IT A FEATHER-LIGHT TOUCH. SLOW YOURSELF DOWN AND MEET THE WORLD OF INTEROCEPTION.

GO EVEN LIGHTER. KEEP CONTACT - THAT'S IMPORTANT - BUT IMAGINE YOUR HANDS FLOATING ABOVE YOUR THIGHS.

WHAT ELSE DO YOU NOTICE? MAYBE YOU GET A SENSE OF WHOLE LEGS, WHOLE SIDES, YOUR HEART AND BREATH. ALIVENESS. PULSING.

THIS IS ME RIGHT NOW, THIS IS MY BODY RIGHT NOW.

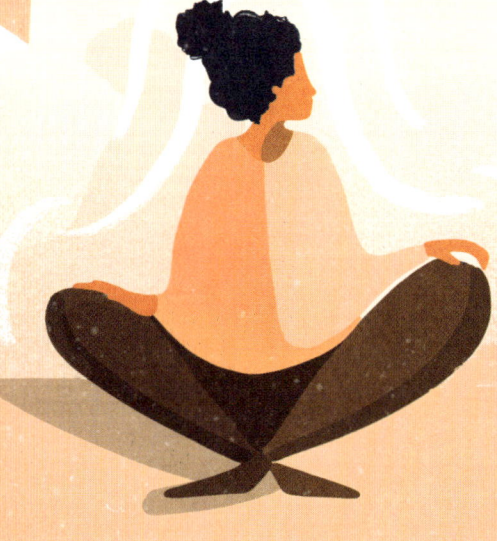

SLOWLY GO BACK TO HEAVY HANDS. IF YOUR PERCEPTION OF YOURSELF CHANGED, MAYBE SOME STRANGE SHAPES AND FEELINGS, EXCELLENT. YOU ARE TUNING INTO THE SLOW BACKGROUND TONE OF YOUR BODY. BE AWARE: IT CAN BE WEIRD IN THERE.

The philosopher Husserl built a whole edifice of knowing based on the 'toucher touching themselves'. Rather that the Cartesian 'I think therefore I am', Husserl offered touch as the foundation of knowing (Welton 1999). For a bodyworker, that is very, very cool.

You are unique; play with naming sensations to learn how you feel. 'It is not necessary for the representation I make of an object to be similar to the object itself; it is enough if I get the same representation every time I see the object' (Quiroga 2017 quoting the 19th-century polymath Hermann von Helmholtz).

BEING TRAUMA-INFORMED IS UNDERSTANDING THAT OCCASIONALLY EVEN SIMPLE EXERCISES LIKE THE ONE OPPOSITE CAN FEEL ACTIVATING. SOMETIMES EVEN THINKING ABOUT THE BODY OR TOUCH IS TERRIFYING.

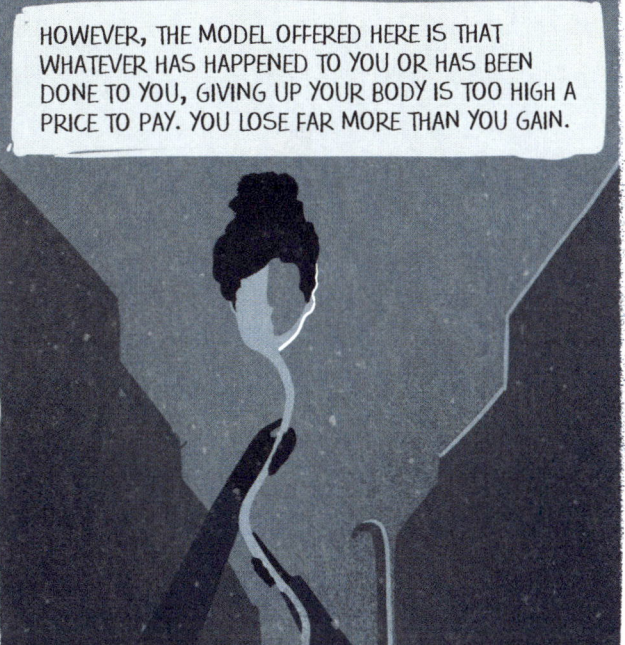

HOWEVER, THE MODEL OFFERED HERE IS THAT WHATEVER HAS HAPPENED TO YOU OR HAS BEEN DONE TO YOU, GIVING UP YOUR BODY IS TOO HIGH A PRICE TO PAY. YOU LOSE FAR MORE THAN YOU GAIN.

IT IS POSSIBLE TO RE-NEGOTIATE TOUCH. MAYBE BY PRACTISING INWARD TOUCH, MAYBE THROUGH SIMPLE GESTURES WITH FRIENDS AND FAMILIES (EVEN OTHER MAMMALS) AND OFTEN WITH A SKILFUL BODYWORKER AS A GUIDE.

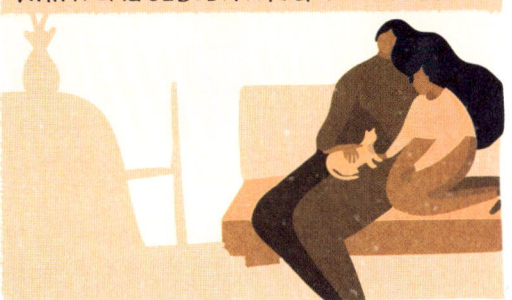

LOOK OUT FOR EARLY SIGNS OF DISTRESS: WE CAN FEEL FLOATY, OUR HANDS OR FEET OR BELLY ARE HARD TO CONTACT, OUR MOUTH IS DRY, OUR THROAT IS TIGHT, OUR BREATH IS HELD, OUR HANDS ARE COLD ON THE CHEEK. THESE ARE SIGNS WE ARE GOING INTO DEFENCE CASCADES OF 'FIGHT-OR-FLIGHT' OR 'FREEZE'.

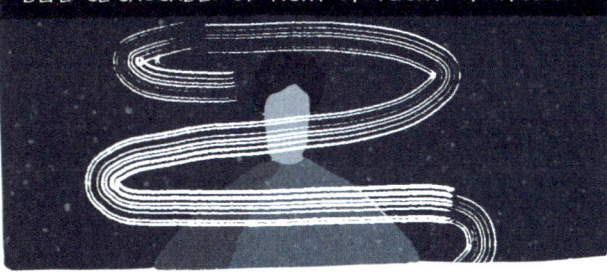

TRY 'OMG' AS 'ORIENT-MOVE-GROUND' TO PUT THE BRAKES ON THE EMERGING CHARGE INSIDE OF YOU.

ALLOW YOURSELF TO WITHDRAW FROM CONTACT TO RE-ESTABLISH SAFETY.

Embodiment is important, but not obvious. Just because we can feel as if our mind is separate from our body, it does not follow that we should encourage the separation. Noë (2006) makes a case for skilful, embodied activity where 'brain, body and world work together to make consciousness happen'.

Any new stimulus that is perceived as safe and meaningful has the potential to shift our physiological state towards health. Most touch is too busy and too focused on local fixes to promote global feelings of safety via interoceptive, inward touch. Slow, relational touch can consistently access primal human needs to be acknowledged, validated and accepted.

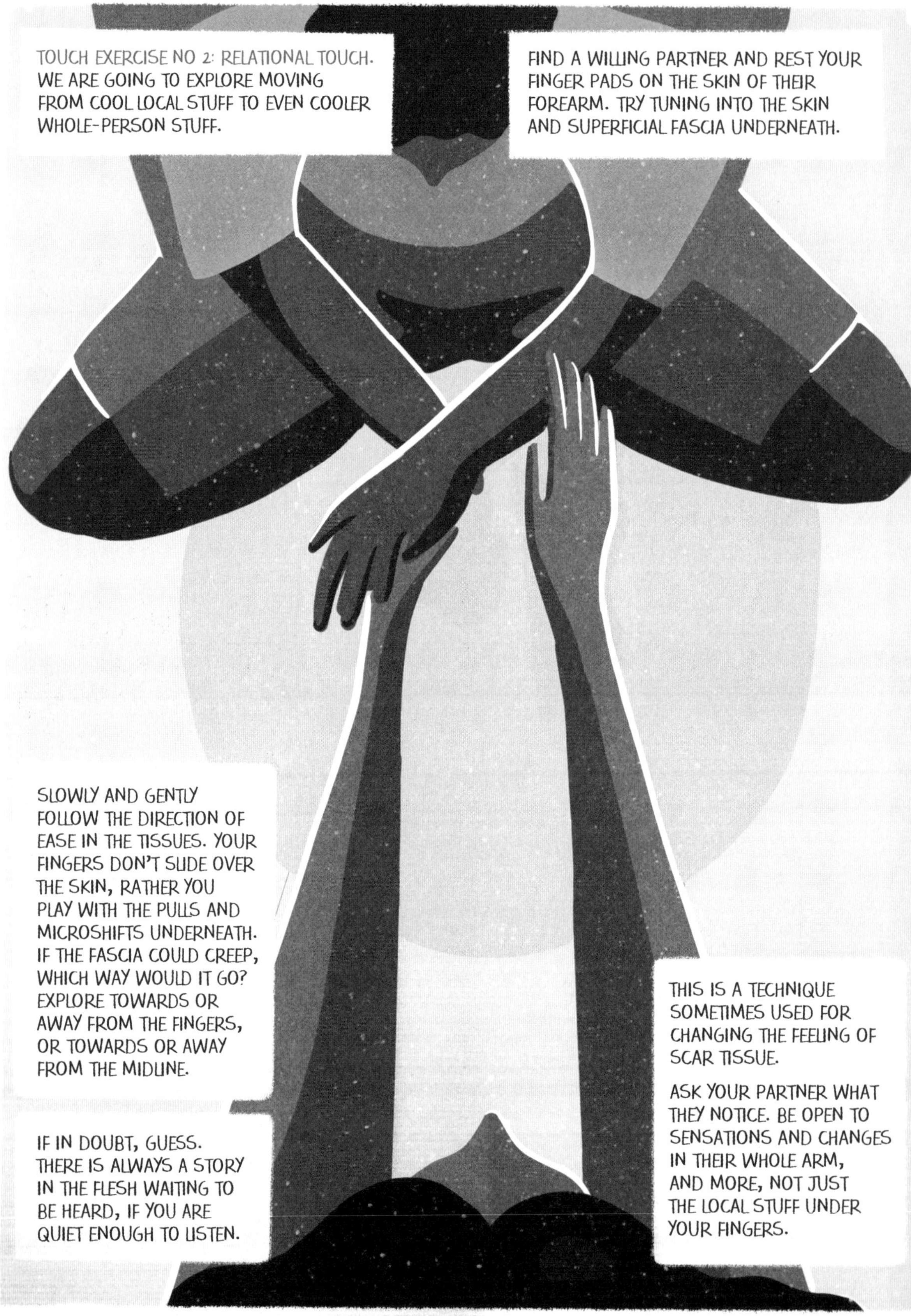
TOUCH EXERCISE NO 2: RELATIONAL TOUCH. WE ARE GOING TO EXPLORE MOVING FROM COOL LOCAL STUFF TO EVEN COOLER WHOLE-PERSON STUFF.
FIND A WILLING PARTNER AND REST YOUR FINGER PADS ON THE SKIN OF THEIR FOREARM. TRY TUNING INTO THE SKIN AND SUPERFICIAL FASCIA UNDERNEATH.
SLOWLY AND GENTLY FOLLOW THE DIRECTION OF EASE IN THE TISSUES. YOUR FINGERS DON'T SLIDE OVER THE SKIN, RATHER YOU PLAY WITH THE PULLS AND MICROSHIFTS UNDERNEATH. IF THE FASCIA COULD CREEP, WHICH WAY WOULD IT GO? EXPLORE TOWARDS OR AWAY FROM THE FINGERS, OR TOWARDS OR AWAY FROM THE MIDLINE.
IF IN DOUBT, GUESS. THERE IS ALWAYS A STORY IN THE FLESH WAITING TO BE HEARD, IF YOU ARE QUIET ENOUGH TO LISTEN.
THIS IS A TECHNIQUE SOMETIMES USED FOR CHANGING THE FEELING OF SCAR TISSUE.
ASK YOUR PARTNER WHAT THEY NOTICE. BE OPEN TO SENSATIONS AND CHANGES IN THEIR WHOLE ARM, AND MORE, NOT JUST THE LOCAL STUFF UNDER YOUR FINGERS.

NOW WE ARE GOING TO MAKE A RADICAL SHIFT.

SETTLE DOWNWARDS INTO YOUR FEET, MOVE BACK INTO YOUR SPINE AND SLOW YOUR BREATH.

BEGIN TO APPRECIATE THE PERSON ATTACHED TO THE ARM. THEY HAVE ALWAYS BEEN THERE, BUT ARE OFTEN FORGOTTEN. THE INTERESTING LOCAL CHANGES DISTRACT US FROM THE BIGGER PICTURE.

THIS PERSON HAS HOPES AND DREAMS AND FEARS. MEET THEM.

HOW OPEN CAN YOU BE? HOW MUCH SAFETY CAN YOU COMMUNICATE VIA YOUR STILL HAND AND STILL PRESENCE? MAYBE BE AVAILABLE FOR EYE CONTACT AND BE BRAVE ENOUGH TO HOLD THE SPACE FOR A COUPLE OF MINUTES.

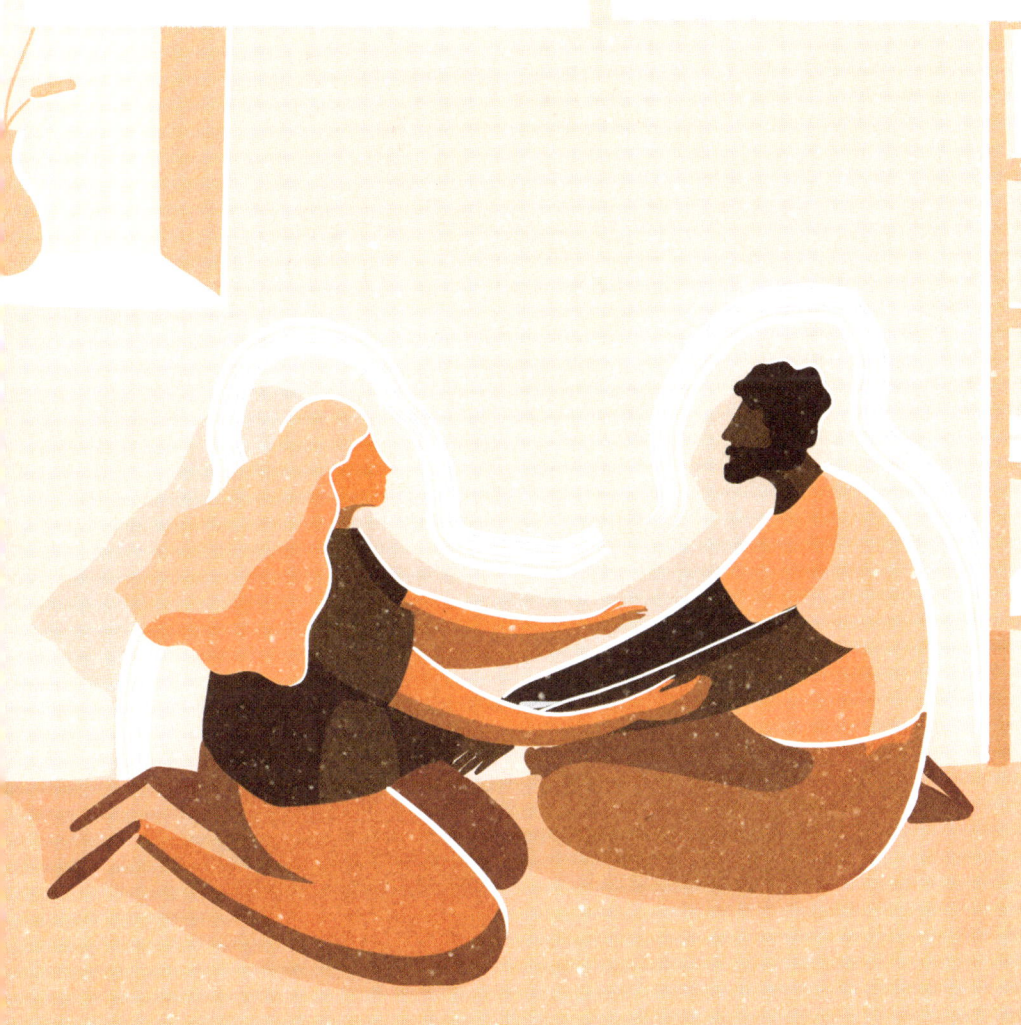

THIS IS RELATIONAL TOUCH. A DIFFERENT, MORE AMBITIOUS, PARADIGM.

TOUCH EXERCISE NO 3: CREATIVE RESISTANCE. FIND A WILLING PARTNER. TRY TO MAKE THIS A PLAYFUL GAME OF GIVING AND RECEIVING RESISTANCE.

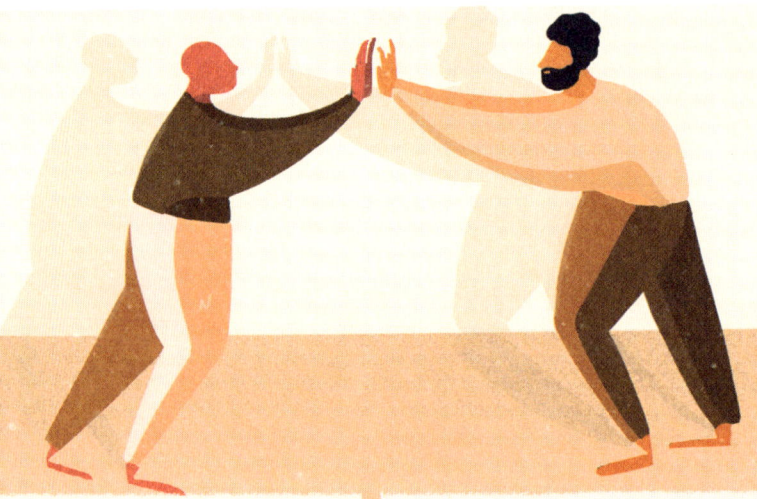

STANDING OPPOSITE YOUR PARTNER, PUT YOUR HANDS UP. ALLOW YOUR PARTNER TO LEAN INTO YOU WITH THEIR HANDS, BUT WITH JUST 20% OF THEIR WEIGHT AND/OR POWER.

OFFER SUPPORT, VERBAL ENCOURAGEMENT AND RESISTANCE. LOTS OF EYE CONTACT AND SMILING FOR 30 SECONDS TO A MINUTE. PAUSE AND ASK THEM TO FEEL THE AFTERGLOW OF THE ACTIVITY.

TRY AGAIN, BUT THIS TIME ENCOURAGE YOUR PARTNER TO BE A BIT MORE ACTIVE, UP TO 50% OF THEIR POWER. PROVIDE ENOUGH RESISTANCE SUCH THAT THEY CAN FEEL THEIR STRENGTH AND POWER.

AFTER 30 SECONDS TO A MINUTE, PAUSE AND REFLECT. IF IT FEELS SAFE IN THE PAUSE, TRY AGAIN. BUILD UP THEIR POWER AND YOUR CREATIVE RESISTANCE; GET THEM TO PUSH YOU BACKWARDS.

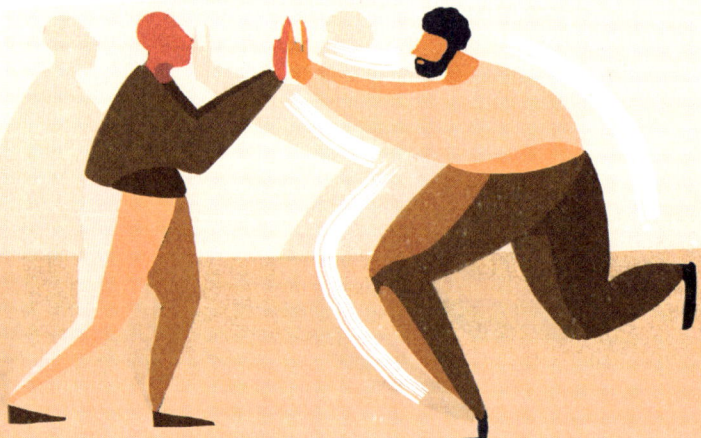

THE GOLDEN RULE IS THE PUSHER ALWAYS WINS, BUT THEY HAVE TO WORK. IN THAT WORK, MANY PEOPLE FEEL AN ALIVENESS AND IGNITION INSIDE OF THEMSELVES. THE OVERCOMING OF RESISTANCE CAN BE A CELEBRATION OF AGENCY AND STRENGTH.

Touch Exercise No 2: Scar tissue technique - see Chaitow and DeLany (2000).
Touch Exercise No 3: There are many ways to use the principle of creative resistance. Lying flat on a massage table, the receiver can slowly straigthen an arm or leg against increasing resistance from the giver.

Clients who are dissociated can be encouraged to do micromovements of pushing their own limbs into a chair or couch and then paying attention to the afterglow of the activity. Brains evolved to move, micromovements often generate a much quicker and easier sense of embodiment than reaching down with the mind alone.

TOUCH EXERCISE NO 4: BRUSHING. THIS IS PROBABLY THE SIMPLEST OF THE TOUCH EXERCISES IN THIS BOOK, BUT YOU GET AN AMAZING PAYOFF OF ENHANCED EMBODIMENT FOR A VERY SIMPLE INTERVENTION.

GET A WILLING PARTNER TO LIE DOWN. GOING SLOWLY AND GENTLY, CUP YOUR HANDS AROUND THEIR SHOULDER AND, WITH A SIMPLE, GENEROUS, LIGHT-TO-MEDIUM CONTACT, BRUSH DOWN THE WHOLE ARM AND OFF THE FINGERS.

HOW MUCH WEIGHT AND SPEED? THE PERFECT AMOUNTS! PRACTISE, GET FEEDBACK AND BE PLAYFUL. REPEAT 3 TO 4 TIMES ON ONE ARM AND THEN REPEAT ON THE LEG ON THE SAME SIDE.

WHEN YOU HAVE DONE ONE SIDE, PAUSE AND ASK THE RECEIVER TO DESCRIBE HOW THE BRUSHED SIDE FEELS COMPARED TO THE UNBRUSHED SIDE. ENCOURAGE YOUR PARTNER TO REALLY LABEL AND EXPLORE THE DIFFERENT SENSATIONS.

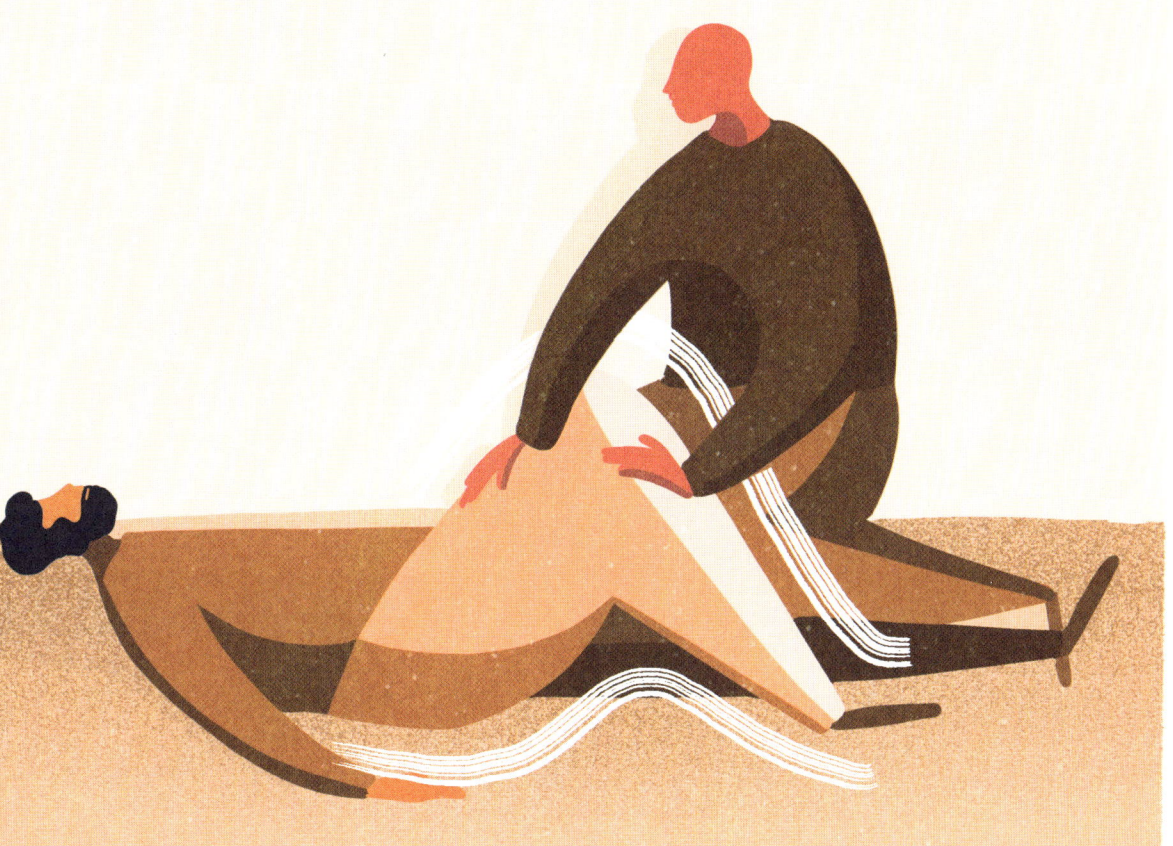

NEARLY ALWAYS THERE IS A DELICIOUS BURST OF GOOD NEWS FROM THE BRUSHED SIDE. AN ENHANCED ALIVENESS AND CONNECTION. DON'T LEAVE THEM HANGING: COMPLETE ON BOTH SIDES - MAYBE EVEN A SIMPLE BRUSHING UNDER THE NECK AND OVER THE SCALP AS WELL.

Finding words for feelings matters. It is a central tenet of the constructed emotion model. By building our vocabulary for nuance and granulations in feeling states we promote more choice, emotional freedom and health (Barrett 2017).

Dissociation is very common. Meeting our bodies is transformational. The skill of embodiment can be a phase shift, like riding a bike; once learnt it is always possible. However, after the phase shift, we need constant practice and support to keep the skill of feeling, more like a tennis serve that needs constant practice to be effective.

WE SHOULD NOT THINK OF TOUCH WORKING BY CHANGING LOCAL TISSUE DYNAMICS. THERE IS MUCH MORE GOING ON. TOUCH CAN HELP US RECONNECT TO, AND IN SOME CASES CHANGE, PRIMAL EXPERIENCES OF HOW WE CREATED OUR SENSE OF SELF.

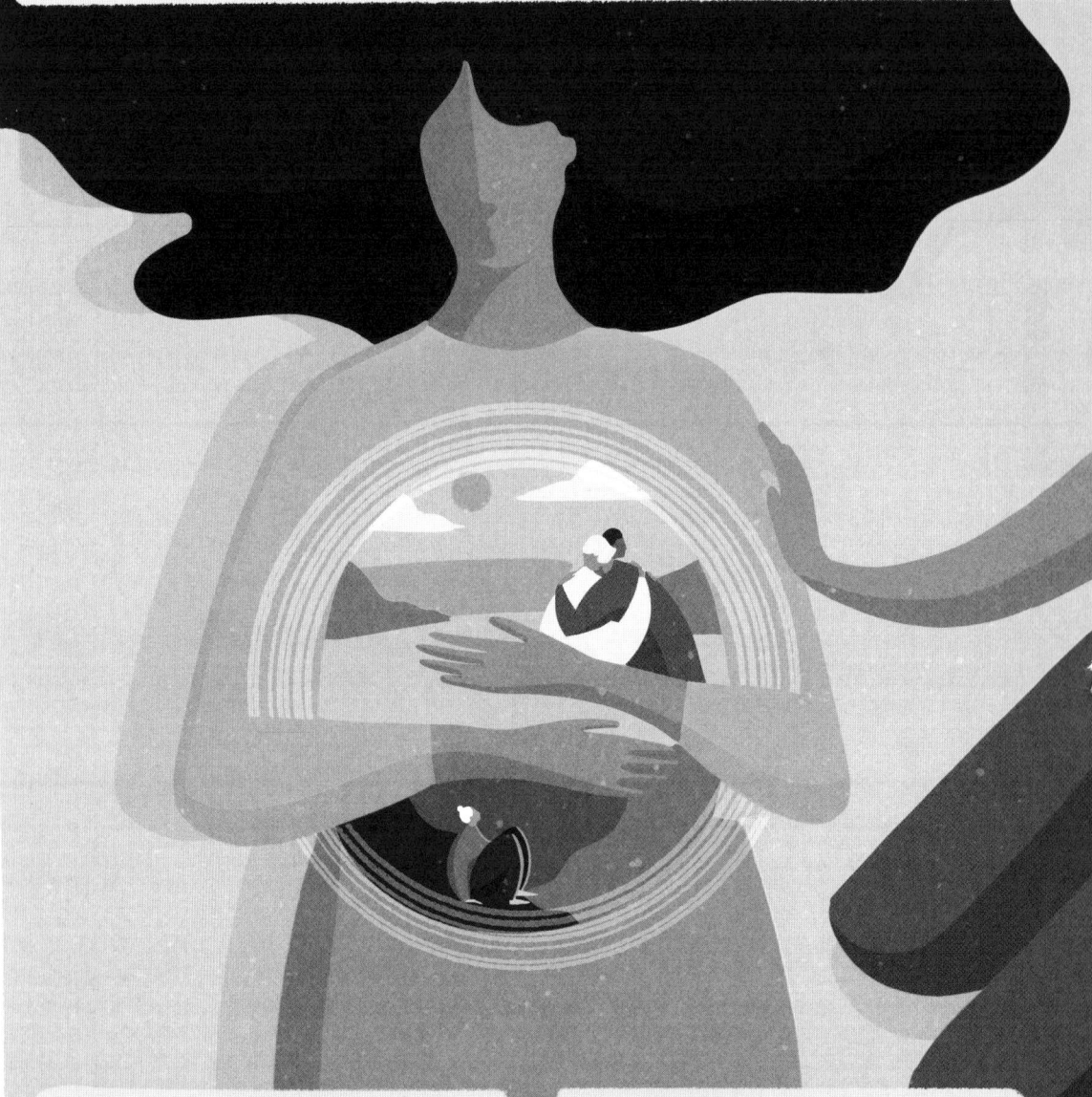

STATEMENTS SUCH AS 'I HAVE TO' OR 'I CAN'T' ARE OFTEN IMPERATIVES FROM EARLY SURVIVAL STRATEGIES EMBEDDED IN OUR BODIES. IN TRAUMA, PAIN AND ANXIETY, TOUCH CAN BE A SAFE, NOVEL STIMULUS TO ACCESS NEW POSSIBILITIES IN OUR PHYSIOLOGY.

TOUCH CAN HELP US MEET OUR WORDLESS PLACES IN A WAY THAT IS HARD TO ACCESS THROUGH CONVERSATION ALONE.

TOUCH IS STRANGER AND MORE POWERFUL THAN OFTEN ASSUMED. WE CAN LEARN TO BE MORE SKILFUL AS WE TOUCH INWARD AND TOUCH OUTWARD.

FEELINGS THAT ARE HABITUALLY SCARY CAN BE RE-FRAMED AND TRANSCENDED.

SLOW, RELATIONAL TOUCH CAN HELP US SHIFT OUR EMOTIONAL CORE AND RELEASE US TO FEEL ALIVE AND CONNECTED.